D1400368

Springer Series: THE TEACHING OF NURSING

Series Editor: Rita R. Wieczorek, PhD, RN, FAAN

1977 Curriculum Evaluation: Theory and Practice
J.L. Green and J.C. Stone *O.P.*

1977 Perspectives on Clinical Teaching: Second Edition
D.W. Smith *O.P.*

1978 Classroom Skills for Nurse Educators
C.C. Clark *O.P.*

1979 Education for Gerontic Nursing
L.M. Gunter and C.A. Estes O.P

1979 The Nurse as Continuing Educator
C.C. Clark *O.P.*

1981 Clinical Experiences in Collegiate Nursing Education: Selection of Clinical Agencies
J.W. Hawkins *O.P.*

1981 Curriculum Development from a Nursing Model: The Crisis Theory Framework
M.B. White, Editor *O.P.*

1984 Teaching Primary Care Nursing: Concepts and Curriculum for Expanded Roles
L.C. Jones *O.P.*

1987 The Nurse As Group Leader: Second Edition
C.C. Clark

1987 Linking Nursing Education and Practice: Collaborative Experiences in Maternal-Child Health
J.W. Hawkins and E.R. Hayes, Editors

1989 A Nuts-And-Bolts Approach to Teaching Nursing
V. Schoolcraft

1990 Educating RNs for the Baccalaureate: Programs and Issues
B.K. Redman, and J.M. Cassells

1991 The Nurse Educator in Academia: Strategies for Success
T.M. Valiga and H.J. Streubert

1993 An Addictions Curriculum for Nurses and Other Helping Professionals: Vol. 1—The Undergraduate Level
E.M. Burns, A. Thompson, and J.K. Ciccone, Editors

1993 An Addictions Curriculum for Nurses and Other Helping Professionals: Vol. 2—The Graduate Level
E.M. Burns, A. Thompson, and J.K. Ciccone, Editors

1993 A Down-to-Earth Approach to Being A Nurse Educator
V. Schoolcraft

1994 The Nurse As Group Leader: Third Edition
C.C. Clark

1995 Teaching Nursing in the Neighborhoods: The Northeastern University Model
P. Matteson

Peggy S. Matteson, PhD, RNC, is an Assistant Professor in the College of Nursing at Northeastern University. Certified as a women's health nurse practitioner, Dr. Matteson's practice and research interests focus on women's health. Since September 1991, as part of her teaching responsibilities she has been working with undergraduate students and collaborating with providers and residents in the neighborhood of Codman Square of Dorchester, MA. She also teaches graduate students within the primary care specialty. During the past 2 years Dr. Matteson's expertise in women's health and the providers' identified needs of the women served by the Codman Square Community Health Center have resulted in three joint research endeavors. Within the College of Nursing Dr. Matteson has served on both the undergraduate and graduate curriculum committees.

Teaching Nursing in the Neighborhoods

The Northeastern University Model

Peggy S. Matteson, PhD, RNC

Editor

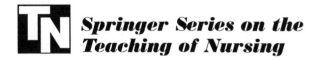

Springer Series on the Teaching of Nursing

Springer Publishing Company, Inc.
536 Broadway
New York, NY 10012

Cover design by Tom Yabut
Production Editor: Pamela Lankas

95 96 97 98 99 / 5 4 3 2 1

Library of Congress Cataloging-in-Publication Data

Teaching nursing in the neighborhoods : the Northeastern University
   model / Peggy Matteson, editor
      p.   cm.—(Springer series, the teaching of nursing)
   Includes bibliographical references and index.
   ISBN 0-8261-9100-2
   1. Nursing—Study and teaching.   2. Community health nursing—
Study and teaching.   I. Matteson, Peggy.   II. Series: Springer
series on the teaching of nursing.
   [DNLM: 1. Education, Nursing.   2. Curriculum.   3. Community Health
Services.   4. Models, Nursing.   W1 SP685SG 1995 / WY 18 T2525 1995]
RT73.T35   1995
610.73'071'55—dc20
DNLM/DLC
for Library of Congress   95-34948

Printed in the United States of America

To the students, faculty members, and community partners who assisted and challenged us to make changes in nursing education, and to Eileen Zungolo, our dean and visionary leader.

Contents

Contributors

Mary Anne Gauthier, EdD, RN, is an Assistant Professor in the College of Nursing at Northeastern University. Certified as a gerontological nurse practitioner, Dr. Gauthier's practice and research interests focus on the meeting the health care needs of the elderly.

Since September of 1991, Dr. Gauthier has served as course coordinator in the first clinical course of the curriculum. As a clinical instructor she works with undergraduate students and collaborates with providers and residents in neighborhoods of Roxbury and Dorchester, MA. She also teaches graduate students within the primary care specialty. Within the College of Nursing Dr. Gauthier has served on the Curriculum Committee providing leadership as co-chair, the Undergraduate Academic Standing Committee, and the Faculty Development Committee.

Barbara R. Kelley, EdD, RN, MPH, CPNP, is an Assistant Professor at the College of Nursing at Northeastern University. Dr. Kelley's practice and research is concerned with cultural diversity. She has spent many years working with culturally diverse and undeserved populations both in the United States and abroad.

At Northeastern University, Dr. Kelley's teaching duties include clinical teaching for the undergraduate students in the neighborhood of East Boston, as well as teaching theory and practicum to graduate students in primary care. She has served as chair of the curriculum committee. Dr. Kelley utilizes her cultural care knowledge and expertise teaching a graduate course in clinical diversity in nursing care. She maintains her clinical expertise as a pediatric nurse practitioner at the Chelsea Health Center pediatric and adolescent clinic in Chelsea, MA.

Margaret Ann Mahoney, PhD, RN, CS, is an Assistant Professor in the College of Nursing of Northeastern University and serves as a coordinator with the Center for Community Health, Education, Research, and Service (CCHERS). As a CCHERS coordinator, Dr. Mahoney works with course coordinators in the College of Nursing and CCHERS coordinators from the neighborhood health centers to organize the community clinical activities for all nursing students and keep the lines of communication open among the partners. She also conducts orientations about neighborhood based clinical experiences for each new class of students and course faculty.

Dr. Mahoney's specialty area is community health nursing and she has helped to shape the health promotion and disease prevention curriculum for the community experiences. In her faculty role she teaches public health to the RN to MS students and advanced practice nursing in the graduate community health program.

Patricia Maguire Meservey, PhD, RN, is an Associate Professor in the College of Nursing at Northeastern University and a Clinical Assistant Professor in the Department of Socio-Medical Sciences at Boston University School of Medicine. In 1991, Dr. Meservey assumed leadership of the Center for Community Health , Education, Research, and Service (CCHERS) as the Executive Director. CCHERS, as consortium of academic institutions and community health centers, is funded by the W.K. Kellogg Foundations and serves as the catalyst for educational reform at the College of Nursing at Northeastern University and School of Medicine at Boston University.

Dr. Meservey's responsibilities for CCHERS and the College of Nursing have encompassed curricula changes, community organizing, interdisciplinary advancements, and policy changes. She has engaged in several studies on the cost of health professions education in community sites and the development of leaders with community health care.

Carole A. Shea, PhD, RN, CS, FAAN, is the Associate Dean for Academic Affairs and Graduate Director in the College of Nursing at Northeastern University. Certified as a Clinical Specialist in Adult Psychiatric and Mental Health Nursing. Dr. Shea's practice and research interests focus on nursing education, mental health policy, and coping with chronic illness.

With more than 20 years of experience in academic teaching, program development, and administration. Dr. Shea has specialized in developing new pathways for nursing education on both the undergraduate and graduate levels. In addition to the nursing curriculum, she has worked with the partners of the Center for Community Health, Education, Research, and Service to develop an interdisciplinary curriculum and community based learning experiences for health professions students.

Eileen Zungolo, EdD, RN, has been Professor and Dean of the College of Nursing at Northeastern University since 1989. She has been an active participant in the development of the Center for Community Health, Education, Research, and Service from its inception. Dr. Zungolo served as the first chair of the Board of Directors of the Center for Community Health, Education, Research, and Service for the maximum time allowed under the by-laws. She currently serves as the vice-chair of the Board.

Dr. Zungolo has advocated curriculum reform and has encouraged faculty definition of their role in the evolution of community based primary care education. She has over 20 years experience in higher education in nursing as a faculty member and administrator.

Foreword

Teaching Nursing in the Neighborhoods: The Northeastern University Model has significance for the field because it brings forward new applied knowledge from a successful model of community-based nursing education. Dissemination of practical knowledge from models that are being built with hard and conscientious work affords health professionals, community leaders, and decision makers the opportunity for wise action based on documented experience. The hour is upon us when the organization of services has begun to change whether or not we are ready. The lack of preparedness for change prevalent in American health services means that change may not take the form—nor work the good—that it would have if it had been undertaken with forethought and attention. Thus, dissemination of information on innovative models is a critical function in the leadership of change.

This book describes the community-based clinical nursing education model developed by the Northeastern University College of Nursing, in partnership with Boston's Center for Community Health Education, Research, and Service (CCHERS). It offers practical guidance for forward-thinking nurse educators who wish to respond to emerging trends by innovating community-based learning for students. The Boston center is one of seven consortia around the country supported by the W. K. Kellogg Foundation in its initiative for Community Partnerships for Health Professions Education.

STRATEGIES FOR BUILDING INTEGRATED, COMPREHENSIVE HEALTH CARE SYSTEMS

The W. K. Kellogg Foundation's health goal is to help people improve their health and that of their communities by building comprehensive, integrated health systems. In these systems four sectors come together: communities, institutions, services, and education. The Community Partnerships for Health Professions Education initiative, of which CCHERS is a part, is one of several strategies designed to work together to bring models of comprehensive, integrated health systems into being.

In formulating the current goal, we at the Kellogg Foundation drew on lessons learned under a 1986 goal. This earlier goal had been devised to shift the paradigm to communities and away from institutional dominance. We thought community-based demonstration projects targeting underserved communities and vulnerable populations were the desirable level for systems change. Our reasoning was that communities that solved high-priority health problems would build upon that success and go on to address and resolve other issues.

Today, our paradigm is the community-institutional partnership. Three lessons from programming under the 1986 goal matured our thinking into the partnership paradigm and the concept of integrating the sectors of communities, institutions, education, and services.

First, we saw that some community-based projects evolved into greater comprehensiveness of service or inclusiveness of those served. This capacity suggested the potential for movement on a continuum from a single- or problem-focus to system building.

Second, we learned that, although the distance between communities and institutions is immense, communities need the institutions' resources and expertise. The chasms are wide, but partnerships can build bridges. An East Baltimore pastor who once asked a Johns Hopkins University researcher recruiting subjects for a study, "Why should we help you when Hopkins just uses neighborhood people as guinea pigs in experiments?" more recently said, "Hopkins was used to coming out in the community and telling us. Now they realize that the community has something to share" (Cohen, 1992).

Third, we learned that strong community-based health service projects did not, on their own, reach the stage of integrating health professions education into service delivery, although they needed to. The Community Partnerships for Health Professions Education initiative grew out of this realization. Health professionals need new models of delivering services through multidisciplinary teams in community sites. For professionals to be available to *practice* in new models, new models have to be available for them to *train* in.

REMEMBERING OURSELVES

Professionals in any field seeking to shape change may see the risk of being overwhelmed by it instead and ask, "Where can we anchor ourselves?" The answer, which nursing is the profession preeminently qualified to give, is to anchor oneself in the worth of the human being. Nursing has the traditions and the values to fight for the worth of the human being. This is the target to keep our eyes on. Knowing the worth of oneself, of the work one does, and of each other person lights the fires of systems change.

The National League for Nursing's vision of the centrality of the consumer in the process of caring is heady stuff. The League's 1993 *Vision for Nursing Education* refers to a "growing consensus between consumers and the nursing community regarding health care reform . . . to serve the health needs of . . . people" (p. 5) and to the role of the consumer as an "informed participant in decisions affecting . . . care" who replaces "hospitals and other institutions" as "the central focus or dominant influence" (p. 6) in the health care system. What would a system look like that the consumer experienced as comprehensive and unfragmented, seamless and user-friendly? This vision contrasts with today's reality, which will not die easily, that the patient is an excuse for grand buildings, professional prestige and prerogatives, technological wizardry, and elite subcultures.

Teaching Nursing in the Neighborhoods is an example of nursing's initiative to value the consumer. Drawing on the CCHERS project's experience in community partnerships, the book intends to guide nurse educators in establishing linkages with communities. Fortunately, today a new literature of applied knowledge is emerging that can strengthen nursing in its pathfinding to new organizational arrangements that affirm the primary value of the person, the family, and the community. *Building Communities from the Inside Out,* a recent work by John P. Kretzmann and John L. McKnight (1993) of the Center for Urban Affairs and Policy Research at Northwestern University, offers a way of viewing and experiencing communities as centers of strength, not regions of deficit. The authors contrast mapping communities in the traditional way, which profiles needs, problems, and deficits, with a new way of mapping. In the new way, resources, assets, strengths, and capacities are profiled.

Future trends disclose that tomorrow's worker will have to have confidence in self and competence in independent decision making. For nursing educators, the task of fostering these attributes is where the practical and the noble converge. Nursing education must foster self-esteem and affirm the student nurse's worth through every means available, or it will fail to prepare professionals of the caliber needed by the health system of the future.

Nursing is up against a very tough task. It is not just a matter of shaping the new. It is a matter of countering forces that would shape the new in nonbenign ways and of countering our habits and what we may have been insidiously taught to think of ourselves. New thoughts will not think themselves. We have to think them. But when we do, our leading thoughts bring new forces into the world to shape it. It is *our power to shape the world* that we must be conscious of and courageously carry forward for the sake of the human. We must cultivate our inner resources, however untested and undeveloped when we begin, to build up the strength for the task in health care reform that the NLN (1993) *Vision* statement reminds us nurse providers must undertake: "to radically redefine their clinical practice, loyalties, political allies, and power nexus" (pp. 6–7). By offering nurse educators an innovative model for reconfiguring clinical education, *Teaching Nursing in the Neighborhoods* is a resource for positive change in health care.

GLORIA R. SMITH, RN, PhD, FAAN
Coordinator of Health Programs and
Program Director at the W. K. Kellogg Foundation
Battle Creek, MI

REFERENCES

Cohen, M. (1992, October). And a neighborhood shall lead them. *Baltimore Magazine*, p. 13.

Kretzmann, J. P., & McKnight, J. L. (1993). *Building communities from the inside out: A path toward finding and mobilizing a community's assets.* Evanston, IL: Northwestern University.

National League for Nursing. (1993). *A vision for nursing education.* New York: Author.

Preface

Clinical learning constitutes the very heart of nursing education. The care students learn to provide and how they come to view their role within the health care system is dependent in part on the clinical learning experiences of their academic program. Traditionally, clinical education occurred almost exclusively within hospitals. Students learned how a community functioned and the nurse's role in that arena during the community health course in the senior year of a baccalaureate program, usually as a final course.

Currently, considerable encouragement is being offered to nursing education programs to broaden the emphasis on clinical education from just inpatient settings to community locales. Although much discussion and attention is being given to the idea of such restructuring, few concrete examples have appeared in the literature to guide this process.

During the past 4 years the faculty of the College of Nursing at Northeastern University in Boston has worked to develop extensive educational experiences in community settings. This book describes how we developed a primary care, community-based approach in a baccalaureate program in nursing. In addition to an overview of the model, this book offers specific illustrations of how clinical faculty developed learning experiences in nontraditional sites. Essentially, the school moved from a curriculum in which most of the students' clinical experiences occurred in the acute care setting to one in which 50% of clinical experiences may take place in the community.

The book should be of interest to anyone involved in nursing or the expanding dimensions of health care. With the direction of health system changes, the book will be most helpful to faculty who are trying to develop a stronger community base within the curriculum and will provide guidance in the refinement of community-based learning activities. Although the focus is on the education of professional nurses at the baccalaureate level, any educator can profit from the insights related to developing community relations and identifying learning activities.

In the development of this curriculum some fundamental beliefs have formed the philosophical foundation of the program:

1. *Nursing students learn about the multiple aspects of a neighborhood and build relationships with residents and providers by returning to the same area for clinical placements across the curriculum.* Initially, this approach was adopted in response to a direct request from the communities. Residents refused to consider having students use a site for a short educational experience and then leave. They wanted students to care about the communities they were learning in and become invested in the well-being of the residents. Such longitudinal assignments have enabled students to develop a sense of connectedness and longitudinal views of health maintenance, health care, and health services, and to experience the reciprocal interface that may only develop over time.

2. *Neighborhood residents and health care providers collaborate with the college of nursing and share in the educational process of its students.* A partnership exists between the students and the residents of a neighborhood. The residents of the neighborhood become shareholders in the students' learning, just as the students are shareholders in the health and well-being of the community they serve.

3. *The collaborative process provides an opportunity for community residents and the academic participants to learn more about the realities of each other's worlds.* Interaction with the members of the neighborhood allows for flexibility and creativity and the variety of opportunities for health care intervention. Rich learning experiences occur as the shackles of "should" are replaced with the freedom and wonder of "could." The variety of possible experiences and potential teachers enables students to feel useful and competent from the first day of clinical education.

4. *Client-centered health care, developed in this collaborative process, empowers both the nursing students and the residents of the neighborhood to become involved in interventions.* Nursing care will incorporate

health promotion and disease prevention, along with acute and chronic care for individuals, families, and the neighborhood as a whole.

5. *Students learn to view health/illness as part of the total lived experience of their clients.* Participation in neighborhood-based programs enables students to learn about the impact of health problems across generations of a family and the neighborhood as a whole.

The changing environment of health care, the need for changes in the education of health providers, and the development of a community partnerships initiative funded by the W. K. Kellogg Foundation are explored in chapter 1. The authors are able speak from their experiences as two of the primary movers in developing a partnership that laid the foundation for educational change and allowed neighborhood health centers, as full partners in the consortium, to function as academic health centers. Patricia Maguire Meservey is the director of the community partnership consortium, the Center for Community Health Education, Research, and Service (CCHERS). Eileen Zungolo is the dean of the College of Nursing at Northeastern University and for several years also served as chair of the executive board of CCHERS.

In her position as associate dean for academic affairs in the College of Nursing, Carole Shea was responsible for making many of the administrative decisions that allowed the implementation of curriculum change. In chapter 2 she discusses the need for reform in nursing education; the effects of a community-based primary health care approach in this reform; the advantages of community-based education for students, faculty, and the community; and the barriers to successful implementation. The use of a metaphor to compare the differences between learning in traditional inpatient sites (learning to swim in a pool) and broadening the focus to multiple community experiences (learning to swim in the ocean) summarizes the advantages of community-based learning for students, faculty, and residents.

Beyond viewing clinical sites as "laboratories" for student learning, working within a partnership model mandates that all members engage in community activities. Faculty, administrators, and students participate in a variety of activities important to those living within the community, such as community meetings, holiday parties, fund-raising activities and food or clothing drives. The needs of the community and the partnership have equal importance with the needs of the educational program.

The remainder of the chapters are written by faculty members involved in the process of working with neighborhoods to enhance student learning, developing new learning opportunities, and exploring dimensions of community life.

Working together, the faculty developed a repertoire of learning activities in which the students could engage. Because they were assigned to different neighborhoods, each was involved with different agencies, serving populations with different needs and different resources. Joint brain storming, sharing ideas, and applying concepts learned in one agency to another environment contributed to the development of a rich inventory of clinical activities.

When a faculty member is challenged to develop community-based clinical sites, there are methods that facilitate the process and increase the chance of success. Identifying and investigating a neighborhood with which to create an alliance, gaining entry to specific sites within the neighborhood, and then developing long-term collaborative relationships is explained in chapter 3 by Peggy Matteson.

The students' first visit to the neighborhood starts their longitudinal educational experience. In chapter 4, Barbara Kelley outlines the components and necessary participants in the introductory process. Tools and techniques that allow the students to start to explore and understand the neighborhood and its inhabitants are explained.

Beginning students have met educational objectives by developing clinical interactions in collaboration with university faculty, neighborhood health care providers, and residents. In chapter 5, Mary Ann Gauthier provides examples of a number of learning experiences within a neighborhood setting that allow the development of professional nursing skills while simultaneously addressing issues of diversity in health beliefs, cultural diversity, family issues, and the role of members of a multidisciplinary care team.

As nursing students progress in their professional development, they more directly interact with community leaders and professionals from a variety of disciplines. Students explore areas of interest in more depth and not only develop nursing skills in communication, critical thinking, and nursing therapeutics but also become more expert in the care of a certain condition or population. In chapter 6, Margaret Mahoney provides examples of students learning activities in the areas of mental health, reproductive and developmental health, and medical/surgical and rehabilitation care.

Chapter 7 evaluates the impact of the program on its participants. Using a framework that compares actual outcomes with anticipated outcomes for students, faculty, and community participants, the authors are able to present some of the initial ideas in the project as well as suggest ways in which these approaches could have been improved. The unexpected challenges and rewards of the experience are also detailed. The insights that are offered in this context could be most helpful for schools planning to move into the community setting.

What these authors have not presented is the extraordinary manner in which they performed in this project from its inception to the present. The authors, all new to Northeastern's College of Nursing at the beginning of this project, have, in pairs or as a team, tackled each problem or obstacle to the implementation of a community-based care model as it arose. They have cheered each other on with each innovation or progressive strategy and consoled each other when a setback occurred. They have been exceptional role models for students, peers, community residents, and providers and most definitely for administrators, for they have genuinely practiced what they have preached. As they have become immersed in the community of their respective neighborhood's assignments, they have also become immersed and committed to the academic community of which they are a part—the College of Nursing and Northeastern University.

All of us who have been involved with this project have lamented that we did not keep journals of our experiences. In addition to the revolutionary changes that we have spearheaded in our educational program, it is important to recall that these changes occurred in a tumultuous context. Everything about the health care delivery system is radically different from what it was 4 years ago. Although most of us believed that the move to community-based care was inexorable, few of us knew that the changes would occur with such rapidity and sweeping nature. The world of nursing is fundamentally different from what it was a few years ago, and it is unlikely that it will return to its previous state. These changes both helped and hurt the move toward community-based nursing education.

The remarkable decline in inpatient care days and the shifting of employment opportunities has lent credence to the movement of the curriculum and learning experiences to the community, as well as heightened the desirability of this curriculum approach in the eyes of the consumer—our prospective students. The extraordinary changes in the health care system have hurt the curriculum innovation merely by creating too much change, too fast for most faculty, affiliating agencies, and colleagues to systematically incorporate new meanings and new worldviews.

Further, we wish that we had recorded our own learning of the process in which we were engaged. All of the authors agree that we had limited insight into the approaches we should take and the processes that we should use, not to mention the world we would find within our neighborhoods. We deeply appreciate the trust and help our neighborhood partners gave, enabling a joint effort to strengthen our students, our services, ourselves, and our community.

Finally, all of the authors of this book are pioneers, for clearly they have helped to make a new approach a viable alternative to traditional views of nursing education. Most important, however, they are women who have a stake in the future, who believe that the future can be better, and who are not afraid to take a chance to make it so. To give the next generation of nurses a broader view of health and the role of nursing in the promotion of health and the prevention of illness, to provide our students with the opportunity to bring all their talents to bear on the improvement of the total life of our patients, and to engage in a genuine partnership with our neighbors as we collectively develop their talents to the fullest—that is what it is all about.

EILEEN ZUNGOLO
Dean, College of Nursing
Northeastern University
Boston, MA

1

Out of the Tower and onto the Streets: One College of Nursing's Partnership with Communities

Patricia Maguire Meservey
Eileen Zungolo

Escalating health care costs and the continual rise in the number of uninsured have drawn the nation's attention to health care reform in the 1990s. Changes will revolutionize the health care system as we know it, creating new roles for health care providers. Northeastern University College of Nursing in Boston has been at the forefront of the change in nursing education through its involvement with the Center for Community Health Education, Research, and Service (CCHERS). The CCHERS, a partnership between academic and community agencies in Boston, was funded by the W. K. Kellogg Foundation to promote the education of health professions students in neighborhood settings. This book describes Northeastern's experience with the program since it was initiated in 1991—the nursing school's curriculum was transformed to provide 50% of its students clinical experience in the community. This chapter reviews the changing environment that requires the shift of health professions education, particularly nursing education, to a community context and summarizes how a collaborative approach contributes to the ability to transform nursing education.

CHANGING ENVIRONMENTS

Over the past 5 years revolutionary changes have occurred in nursing and the health care delivery system. While the news media, talk shows, and editorials have reflected the legislative and political struggles with health care reform in every state, city, and community in the United States, simultaneous alterations in health-related disciplines have occurred. The advent of diagnostic related groups (DRGs) is often noted as a point of departure for the current round of change. The use of DRGs formalized and mandated growing attention to expensive care processes, with hospitalization at the top of that list (Lake, 1992). Although the development of laser surgery and other technologies have reduced the invasive nature of some medical and surgical interventions, shortened length of stays are usually related to early discharge, not to faster recovery rates. Today's hospitals are the site for complex or invasive treatments but not places where patients fully recover.

Other institutions, such as rehabilitation agencies and long-term care facilities, are finding that their patients enter sicker, require more complicated care, and need more skilled nursing attention. Concurrently, the nature and length of patient stay are altered. When patients return home, families, by necessity, are more directly involved and in some cases directly responsible for care. Traditional home health services, such as visiting nurse associations, have a burgeoning patient census, and home care enterprises are emerging. Evidence of the expansion in the home health sector includes an estimated 68% growth since 1981 and projection of an average annual growth rate of 17% for the future (Bowman, 1992).

These events have had an impact on the delivery and cost of health care services. Mounting attention has been focused on analyzing the way in which health care is financed and paid for. Insurance plans, benefits, and the various modes of packaging these items have been scrutinized, and the era of managed care has begun. The identification of domains of care that enhance recovery and speed convalescence is gaining in importance. Consequently, coordination of care, long advocated by nurses, is now receiving increased attention. Nurses who have consistently served in a coordinating role between and among various disciplines find that they hold special knowledge of each professional's plan of care and therefore are excellent managers of a patient's total care needs.

Once nursing determined appropriate management of the ill, it took only a small step to assess the impact these same principles of care would have on those who were well. If health professionals could, in fact, improve a person's recovery through careful planning and teaching about the disease and its management, why not apply the same processes to maintaining health?

Primary care and primary care practitioners are the new buzzwords heard in the media and health care reform rhetoric and appear to point the way to the future. In the past, achieving center stage has not been easy for those invested in primary care. Lacking the "glamour" of acute care and certainly lacking the funding base that hospitals have enjoyed, primary care in community settings has been largely the result of dedicated community members who worked to make health care available in their neighborhoods.

The need for primary care services is increasingly evident in U.S. health statistics. More than 35 million Americans lack health insurance (Shields & Wolfe, 1992). Without this financial support, access to preventive care is jeopardized. As a result, morbidity rates for preventable and readily curable diseases, such as rubeola (54/100,000 under age 15) and syphilis (54/100,000), are escalating (National Association of Community Health Centers, 1993). Likewise, there are skyrocketing increases in illness caused by unhealthy life-styles. The impact of alcohol and drug abuse, smoking, and poor nutrition burdens the health care system with unnecessary illness and costs.

A study conducted by the Commonwealth of Massachusetts Rate Setting Commission (1994) revealed that 1 in every 10 hospital stays in Massachusetts was preventable. The ambulatory care–sensitive conditions (i.e., illness that can be treated in an outpatient setting) were grouped into three categories: avoidable conditions, such as those preventable by immunization or proper nutrition; acute conditions, such as bacterial pneumonia and dehydration; and chronic conditions, such as asthma and hypertension. More timely interventions for these health deviations would have saved the commonwealth $473 million! The significance of inadequate primary care services is intensified when regions of concentrated poverty are analyzed. In the Massachusetts study, the highest preventable hospitalization rates were found in the inner cities, where the poverty rate is substantially greater than the state's average.

Further investigation of the data reveals that disproportionate risk falls on the vulnerable populations of children, elderly, and women. Likewise, the poor, minorities, and migrant workers continue to suffer the highest incidence of preventable and readily treatable illnesses. As the nation examines mechanisms to contain health care costs and overcome the deficiencies of the current system, radical departure from the status quo must occur. Managed care and the concepts of primary and preventive care throughout health and illness are major forces moving the nation toward a system change.

The financial underpinnings of managed care have created an environment in which genuine collaboration is profitable. Because managed care requires comprehensive health services through health and illness, health care agencies are finding it necessary to enter into joint ventures. For example, a typical health maintenance organization (HMO) may provide primary care services, care for common illness, and support services, such as radiology and laboratory. It may not, however, include within its organization an acute care hospital and the specialty service therein. The HMO must negotiate an arrangement with the hospital to provide care to its enrollees. Likewise, the hospital needs the flow of patients to continue its services from a financial perspective and to provide the critical cadre of patients to support quality care from a clinical perspective. The services of the primary and outpatient care must be integrated with the services of inpatient care to minimize fragmentation, duplication, and omissions. Thus, managed care has ramifications far beyond its financial basis. Managed care requires a reconfiguring of the health care system through an integration of services among traditional agencies and professionals. Managed care can best be implemented with the linkage of existing health services into network systems. Partnerships among insurers, community health centers, and hospitals have the potential to promote high quality in the new care mechanism. When educational institutions are added to this mix, the resources of new providers, research opportunities, and the inquisitiveness of scholarship add to the diversity within this partnership and bring the systems to a level of excellence.

HEALTH CARE PARTNERSHIPS

History presents many examples of efforts to create joint projects between academic institutions and communities, government and communities, business and communities, and communities and communities. Most projects have been based on determinations of community needs formulated by people who were external to and not residents of the community. Hence, interventions were often not a genuine reflection of community planning. Settlement houses provide a fine example of this process. Founded most often by affluent women, settlement houses offered a range of services to an immediate neighborhood. The initial focus was to assist people in gaining employment opportunities and the training required to secure a job. Services quickly expanded, however, as it became clear that to sustain gainful employment a person needed to be in good health (primary care) and have care provided for his/her children (day care).

President Lyndon Johnson's Great Society and Model Cities programs built upon the concept of addressing community concerns but used "top down" strategies and mechanisms. Both programs were intended to link community representatives with the government to effect changes within the social fabric on the community. The goal of these programs was to develop opportunity for the low economic groups through job programs, improved environments, and education (Wofford, 1980). The tragic flaw of the programs was their placement in Washington, DC, a de facto loss of the critical connection between the programs, and the communities they intended to serve.

Count Gibson, MD, and Jack Geiger, MD, did not repeat the mistakes of the programs developed by the Johnson administration. Having worked in South Africa, these pioneer physicians returned to the United States with a concept of a community-developed health care system. Gibson and Geiger developed a truly community-based model by asking community groups about their care needs. The outcome of their efforts was two community health centers, Columbia Point in Dorchester, Massachusetts, and Mount Bayou in Mississippi (Young, 1982). Now, more than 1,200 commr nity health centers dot the nation, providing a wide range of health care that encompasses the physical, psychological, social, and economic aspects of wellness.

The health center model is based on the notion of community control. The power to determine services for a community is vested in the community. As such, the board of directors, the governing body of the health center, is composed of community residents. In this type of system health care providers function as consultants, not ultimate decision makers. Collaboration along these lines has produced a delivery system that is responsive to the unique needs of a community and has enjoyed considerable success in inner cities and rural settings.

NURSING EDUCATION

Concurrent with these developments in the community health services, health professions education is also experiencing rapid change. Whereas the rhetoric of health care reform focuses on the presumed effect of a legislated package of change, the reality for consumers and providers is that health care reform is a fait accompli. The impact of reform on the education of health professions is significant. The reduction in patient-care days in an illness episode has led to a restriction in the ways in which student experiences can be organized and offered in a hospital setting. Specifically, the cessation of admissions for diagnostic and preoperative purposes has limited students' ability to obtain a full picture of a person. All too frequently, the student does not have the opportunity to see the patient over any length of time because patients are discharged early in the recovery phase. Consequently, students develop a limited perspective of the course of an illness. Of equal importance, they are unable to build therapeutic relationships with patients because of limited opportunity for continuity in their contacts.

At the same time those patients who endure a hospitalization at exceeds a few days are usually critically ill. Baccalaureate education in nursing aims to prepare the entry-level nurse, and the acute setting does not provide the diversity of learning experiences to fulfill this educational goal. Increasingly, the acute care setting does not offer an adequate range of clinical problems. Of equal concern, changes in acute care settings do not allow the student to spend sufficient time with patients to grasp the concepts underlying recovery and a return to normalcy.

Despite these limitations, the vast majority of nursing and medical education continues to take place in hospital settings. Yet diagnosis of disease, much of treatment, and all but the early part of recovery occur outside the hospital. When students are provided the opportunities for ambulatory care experiences, these are often limited to the outpatient settings of the hospital. These centers usually are structured by specialty practice in an illness-oriented medical model of care. Students do not gain the breadth of knowledge necessary for primary care services, including the continuity of comprehensive patient care. Also absent from this model is the link of the community: public health concerns and the whole range of problems that beset people but are not directly manifested in their physical health. Hospitals and ambulatory care centers present a top-down approach that isolates the patient and fragments care.

In response to this scenario, much of the leadership in nursing education has advocated that nurse educators make a more aggressive move to a community focus. *A Vision for Nursing Education,* a publication by the National League for Nursing (1993), advocates a shift in nursing education to a community-based, community-focused health care system in which health-promotion and disease-prevention strategies are engineered for individuals and communities. Furthermore, with this document, the NLN dramatizes its commitment to the development of new structures and relationships with diverse constituents to develop educational experiences where people work, play, go to school, and live.

To prepare for future practice, students need experiences in neighborhood-based settings. Community health centers, nursing centers, and the neighborhoods in which they are located can provide a depth and breadth of experiences for student learning. Health centers, however, may be hesitant to enter into a teaching relationship. Having provided care to underserved populations, health centers have experienced the abuse of inferior care and opportunistic research. Once burned, they move slowly. Their interest in teaching is found in their foundation of community involvement. Academic institutions seeking affiliations with health centers need to approach them from the orientation of the community and the values of community-based service.

INVOLVEMENT OF PRIVATE FOUNDATIONS

There are several large private foundations that focus their attentions on health care issues and needs. Funding for research studies and educational initiatives often provides health care educators with the stimulus to move toward change. For example, the Pew Charitable Trusts determined that "the education and training of health professionals is out of step with the evolving health needs of the American people" (Pew Health Professions Commission, 1991). A report created by educators, consumers, and interdisciplinary professionals from both the public and the private sectors identified competencies that will be needed by the health practitioners of the future. They predicted that the practitioner in the year 2005 will care for the community's health, expand access to effective care, emphasize primary care, ensure cost-effective services, involve patients in decision making, promote healthy life-styles, and prevent disease.

The W. K. Kellogg Foundation created the Community Partnerships Initiative (CPI), a futuristic educational program designed to transform nursing and medical education. The CPI was developed in response to multiple observations and concerns about the health care system and was in keeping with the overall goal of health planning at the foundation, which aimed at the creation of a coordinated, cost-effective, and comprehensive health care system equally accessible to all people (*Community partnerships*, 1992).

CPI Strategies

Within the CPI, the Kellogg Foundation envisions a transformation of health care firmly based on the community philosophy of Geiger and Gibson. This would entail a change in orientation from a system developed for providers and organizations to one centered on people and communities. The philosophy of the CPI engages communities as full partners in health care and health profession education, assuring the community empowerment with regard to quality determinations. To implement this set of beliefs, change in four critical areas was identified: a reorientation of health professions education, promotion of interdisciplinary care and education, advancement of community-responsive research, and increased accessibility to services.

First, funding was established to reorient health professions education to community-based primary care. The Kellogg Foundation envisioned that educational institutions would be encouraged to work in partnership with communities through the creation of community-based teaching centers. These centers would emphasize primary care in a multidisciplinary model, thus enhancing both education and service. An underlying assumption is that new practitioners will choose a community-based practice if they have been exposed to and socialized into the practice arena in an interdisciplinary learning mode. To be valued by students, community-based primary care must be valued by faculty and given the same emphasis in health professions curricula as is given to institution-based care. Thus, a comparable amount of curricula time and clinical practice must occur in the community setting.

Second, community-based primary care brings health professionals together in interdisciplinary groupings to provide care. Much has been written about the advantages of using teams of various health professionals for the coordination of care. Nonetheless, most of what is practiced is a "turn" care system. For example, the physician sees the patient and develops a medical care plan; nurses then take their turn and develop the nursing care plan; other health professionals do the same, and so on. More frequently than not, these various approaches to addressing patient problems and concerns are not merely unrelated, they are incompatible. Hence, the unique knowledge, autonomy, and independence of professionals can contribute to fragmentation of patient care, undermine interdisciplinary collaboration, and pull professions apart. Each discipline can, theoretically, complete its work in isolation without the knowledge of another group. The reality in health care, however, is multiple professions with overlapping fields of knowledge and a scope of work that requires more that one discipline to complete the tasks. Medicine, nursing, social work, physical therapy, and psychology cannot provide comprehensive health care without support from each other.

The need for multiple professions collaborating in health care has intensified with the complexity of care needed in today's world. Clearly, interdisciplinary services and collaboration are essential to any system of managed care.

Third, as the new system of health care emerges, there is a critical need to investigate its effectiveness and efficiency. Community-responsive research incorporates public health, primary care, and community-based concerns within one integrated domain of knowledge. As health service research has transformed the delivery system, community-responsive research can transform communities. It brings the talents of the scientist to the pragmatic needs of community and can provide a scholarly metamorphosis in the community. Boyer (1991) describes this type of investigation as the Scholarship of Application. Taking knowledge believed to be true, applying the information to practice in the community, and assessing its effectiveness offer scholarship that is of direct use to society.

Finally, large groups of people are not receiving the health care services they need. Within the overall CPI philosophy is a focus on communities in which the residents are especially vulnerable, at high risk, and underserved. Through the community-academic partnership, the community identifies the priority needs, and the faculty and health care providers respond with the knowledge and skill to address them. Such collaboration yields enriched and expanded services to improve the health of the community while increasing the services available and fostering student learning in areas in which the clinical needs are high and new models of health care are emerging.

CPI PROCESS

Noting these changes and needs in health care, the W. K. Kellogg Foundation developed a Request for Proposal (RFP) that ignited the health professions educational groups. Essentially, the RFP mandated a multidisciplinary approach to health professions education, with nursing and medicine at a minimum. Of the 132 schools of medicine in the country, 126 joined forces with a nursing program and other health professional schools and participated, submitting letters of intent. From this original number and after the full proposal development by 15 groups, the Kellogg Foundation selected seven partnership sites to receive grants of $6 million each over 5 years (see Table 1.1). This large allocation of funds awarded by the Kellogg Foundation demonstrates its intent to facilitate a revolutionary change in health professions education.

CPI IN BOSTON

Initial Development

In response to the original request for proposals from the Kellogg Foundation, faculty members from Northeastern University College of Nursing and Boston University School of Medicine and staff from Boston's Department of Health and Hospitals and Codman Square Health Center, a neighborhood health care facility in the Greater Boston area, drafted a letter of intent. In December 1990 the fledgling partnership was funded to participate in a planning year. The Kellogg Foundation had selected 15 of the respondents to the RFP to participate in a planning year that would entail four national meetings of the participants. These meetings were organized to enable the development of the participants in a variety of aspects of community-based initiatives, primary care trends, interdisciplinary education, health professions education issues, and emerging developments in health care reform.

A small corps of faculty, along with Boston's health officials and health center representatives, participated in these meetings and learned much about national and international partnerships. The participants began to envision a partnership between the academic institutions and the existing community health centers in the city. Boston has the greatest concentration of health centers in the country, with 24 health centers serving the city's 600,000 residents. Using a process similar to the one used by the Kellogg Foundation, the Boston "Working Group" (the original name of the CCHERS) contacted the Massachusetts League of Community Health Centers, the state's primary care association, for assistance. In an inclusionary process each of the health centers in Boston was invited to submit a letter indicating its interest and ability to participate in the education of health professionals. The format of this letter was comparable to the initial announcement of the CPI funding opportunity and included the criteria the Kellogg Foundation had originally identified. Using this process, three additional neighborhood health centers were selected. Fac-

TABLE 1.1 Community Partnerships Initiative, W. K. Kellogg Foundation

City, State	Primary Partners
Boston, MA	Center for Community Health Education, Research, and Service: Northeastern University College of Nursing, Boston University School of Medicine Boston's Department of Health and Hospitals, Bowdoin Street Health Center, Codman Square Health Center, Dimock Community Health Center, Dorchester House Multi-Service Center, East Boston Neighborhood Health Center, Harbor Health Services, Inc. Little House Health Center, Mattapan Community Health Center, South Boston Community Health Center, Whittier Street Neighborhood Health Center
Atlanta, GA	Morehouse School of Medicine, Georgia State University School of Nursing, Emory University School of Nursing, Clark Atlanta University School of Social Work, Southeastern Primary Care Consortium
Honolulu, HI	Ke Ola O Hawaii: University of Hawaii Schools of Medicine, Nursing, Social Work, and Public Health; Waianae Coast Comprehensive Health Center; Kalihi-Palama Health Clinic; Queen Emma Clinic; Kokua Kalihi Valley Homes Project; Rural Oahu Family Planning Project
East Lansing, MI	Michigan State University Colleges of Human Medicine, Nursing and Osteopathic Medicine; Kirtland Community College; Thunder Bay Community Health Services; Northern Michigan Health Services
Johnson City, TN	Office of Rural and Community Health: East Tennessee State University Schools of Medicine, Nursing, Public Health, and Allied Health; Mountain City Family Health Center; Extended House Clinic; Rogersville Health Education Center
El Paso, TX	Institute of Community Health Education, University of Texas at El Paso, Texas Tech University, Lower Valley Communities
West Virginia	University of West Virginia Systems: West Virginia University; Health Science Center (Medical, Nursing, Pharmacy, Dental), Marshall University Medicine and Nursing, Rainelle Medical Center, Roane County Health Care Insurance, Cameron Medical Center, Camden-on-Gaulen Medical Center, West Virginia School of Osteopathic Medicine

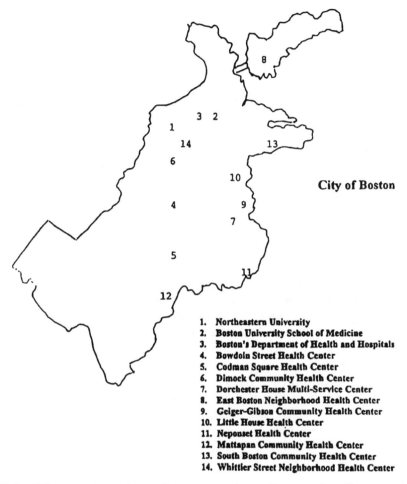

City of Boston

1. Northeastern University
2. Boston University School of Medicine
3. Boston's Department of Health and Hospitals
4. Bowdoin Street Health Center
5. Codman Square Health Center
6. Dimock Community Health Center
7. Dorchester House Multi-Service Center
8. East Boston Neighborhood Health Center
9. Geiger-Gibson Community Health Center
10. Little House Health Center
11. Neponset Health Center
12. Mattapan Community Health Center
13. South Boston Community Health Center
14. Whittier Street Neighborhood Health Center

FIGURE 1.1   Location of partner sites, Center for Community Health Education Research and Service.

tors significant in the selection of specific health centers included their ability to provide meaningful learning experiences for the health profession students, including proximity to educational institutions, physical plant, and client population in terms of cultural diversity and health status. [In fall 1993 eight additional neighborhood health centers joined the partnership through a similar process (see Figure 1.1).]

The Working Group was expanded to include representatives

from each of the neighborhood health centers, the city, and academic institutions. During this phase, the group could best be described as loosely organized. There was a consistent and conscious effort to operate on a principle of inclusion: anyone who wanted to participate in the "project" was encouraged to do so. Consequently, although there was a core of approximately 10 people who worked on a consistent and vigorous basis, many others attended meetings sporadically.

The Working Group recognized that some serious thought needed to be directed toward the values that would form the basis for the project. The group was sensitive to the historical development of the community health centers, which grew out of the need for health care services external to hospital settings and accessible to families. Formerly, the only health care short of hospitalization open to intercity community members was through hospital outpatient departments. Such units were staffed by medical residents (graduate medical students), who received limited supervision from the attending physician, rotated among the various clinical services of the hospital, were not necessarily committed to primary care, and often were oblivious to the needs of families in their communities. Hence, the community health centers emerged with a desire for ownership vested squarely in the hands of the community. itself. Concomitantly, the dissatisfaction with health services that the community had experienced was associated with health professions education. A well-founded skepticism existed regarding health professions, along with a perception that educational institutions used communities when they needed subjects for their studies or patients for teaching their students. Community members saw health professions students as having no understanding of their autonomous authority and no commitment to them.

During this earlier time, members of the academic institutions were remote from and therefore uninformed about developments in the community movement. Health professions educators were heavily vested in the acute care environment, and most assumed that the hospital was the mecca of clinical learning. As a result, they were unaware of the health needs and wealth of learning opportunities in the community. In light of these disparate orientations, the establishment of trust through genuine shared problem solving and open dialogue were indispensable elements of the developing partnership. As members of the Working Group defined the parameters of the project, they began to understand each other's perspective. This remains an ongoing process in which academicians, community health care providers, and community members continue to learn and gain insights about their respective viewpoints and priorities.

Implementation of CPI Strategies and Goals

In accordance with CPI strategies and goals, the health profession schools made a commitment to collaboratively design educational and service opportunities with communities. The primary purposes of this partnership are to create academic health centers in the community for primary care and redirect health professions education into the primary care sector. These goals must be fulfilled with the full participation and involvement of the residents of the communities. Inherent in the philosophy of the CCHERS partnership is the belief that the health services of the community are owned by the community and that the power to direct its health and welfare is the right and responsibility of the community. The community grants permission to the academic programs to participate in the this process with the proviso that the health profession students understand that they are guests in the community. The academic programs are committed to educating students to participate and work with communities in the development of culturally sensitive and comprehensive health care planning. Last, but far from least in these considerations, is an appreciation that to be truly community-based the project has to be embraced and owned by the community.

To achieve these goals a variety of mechanisms were put into place. First, one member of the Working Group from an academic institution was "assigned" to work with each neighborhood health center. In this manner, the academicians could learn firsthand about the centers and, after consultation with community members and health center staff, summarize the potential educational opportunities therein. The faculty member could also begin to establish a working relationship with the community. This representative, in concert with the chief executive officer (who was also a member of the Working Group), made a presentation to the board about the venture to engage in an academically oriented partnership. In each of the four neighborhood health centers the community boards agreed to participate in the project.

Second, open community-based meetings were held and widely publicized to solicit input on the project. Invitations were sent to community-based organizations, health care providers, faculty from multiple health-related disciplines at Boston University and Northeastern University, formal consumer groups, and community members. The meetings were extraordinary in the interest they generated. There was a huge outpouring of interest from the expanded community with attendance of more than 50 people at most meetings and often more than 100.

These information sessions were very helpful in the development of the thinking underpinning CCHERS. For example, it was clear that rotating students through communities was a totally unacceptable idea to the community representatives and reminded them of the transient medical providers of the past that the neighborhood health centers were formed to offset. It was evident that mechanisms were needed to build continuity into the students' learning experiences. Educational experiences were thus designed to provide a longitudinal pattern for student learning. Students begin their clinical learning in a given neighborhood and systematically return to the same community throughout their educational program. As students grow in competence in practice and knowledge of the community, their contributions become substantial. Similarly, to prepare nursing and medical students to function effectively in community-based primary care, it is essential that the community cooperate fully in the enterprise. As a result, the residents of the neighborhoods are direct partners in the education of students, the development of service projects to meet community needs, and the identification of community-responsive research problems.

Third, to achieve goals of partnership and service it became evident that the bulk of the funding from the Kellogg Foundation needed to be funneled to the communities to develop the necessary structure for an academic community-based health center. Further, it seemed critical to demonstrate in the most elementary way possible that the engineers of this project were committed to assuring a level playing field among the partners in the allocation and distribution of funds. Not only did placing the money in the communities dramatically demonstrate the commitment to place the community first, it also clearly communicated the end to "business as usual."

CCHERS Governance

To preserve the community's ownership and cement the relationships, the organizational structure that emerged for the partnership had to be based on equality among the partners and retention of authority within the communities. To this end it was determined that the new organization's name would reflect the partnership and not any one of the institutions in the coalition. The acronym CCHERS highlights the Boston locale and emphasizes the community. The form of governance would be through a board of directors with each "partner" (i.e., Boston's Department of Health and Hospitals, Northeastern University, Boston University, and the four neighborhood health centers) holding two seats on the board. One of the neighborhood health center representatives is a member of the community, not employed by the health center; the second designee is a staff member of the health center. An executive committee is elected from the board and must represent each of the constituents—that is, each academic institution, the neighborhood health center, and the community. (See Figure 1.2.)

The board functions in the same way as a not-for-profit organization, and although not legally incorporated, it is exploring that option. As such, CCHERS has developed bylaws to guide its work, and the board serves as a policy-making body. All policies related to the partnership are determined by the board, as are decisions regarding jointly received funding (i.e., the budget through the Kellogg Foundation).

Standing Committees

There are now four standing committees of the board of directors, created to facilitate the work of CCHERS. Each evolved from the original working group and the logical division of work defined during the model development phase. The four committees are education, research, government affairs, and finance. Each

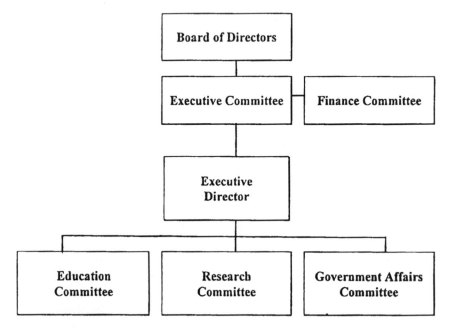

FIGURE 1.2 Governance structure, Center for Community Health Education, Research, and Service.

committee has representation from all three constituents of the partnership: university, health center, and community.

Education Committee

A key responsibility of the Education Committee is faculty development. Within the project, faculty members are defined as participants in the direct education of health professions students and include traditional university faculty, participating providers employed by the health center, community outreach workers and coordinators employed through the project, and contributing members of the community or community-based agencies. Each of the above groups has unique needs, yet common domains have also been identified. Much of the formal emphasis has been to provide educational sessions exploring the core concepts of community-based practice and teaching methodologies. Informally, an ongoing dialogue takes place between and among these groups in role making, role defining, and exploration of ways to enhance the partnership on individual basis.

The Education Committee is also responsible for identifying the common curricular areas across nursing and medicine and the content areas required for community-based practice. Through a collaborative process, core concepts were identified and serve as the guideline for multidisciplinary experiences in the community setting. Some of the discussion at the community meetings mentioned earlier had curriculum issues as a main agenda item. What did the community believe health professionals needed to know to meet community needs? What knowledge and skills did health care providers see as areas that needed strengthening in their educational experience? The neighborhood health center administrators and health care providers had invaluable insights in response to these questions. The Education Committee incorporated these ideas into curriculum guidelines, which have influenced the refinement of curriculum development in the educational institutions. There are also mechanisms for the Education Committee to directly influence the academic institutions' curriculum committees. In its continuing work the Education Committee guides the implementation of the nursing and medical curricula in the community through an ongoing process of planning, evaluation, and redesign.

Research Committee

The Research Committee aims to foster community-responsive research, as advocated by the Kellogg Foundation in the CPI. As noted previously, research of this type is conducted in communities and focused on the needs and concerns of that community. Through the multidisciplinary committee, community needs have been identified and priorities for research delineated. Seasoned researchers from the universities are being recruited to work in collaboration with health center staff and community members in the implementation of research studies. The outcomes are a mix of several different approaches to research development. First, researchers with existing projects that match with community needs are being connected with health centers to expand work in specified areas. Second, where community needs do not immediately match with established research, the committee is moving to identify researchers in related areas to modify their work to meet community needs. Third, the communities and health centers are developing research protocols and processes to facilitate the approval of research within the community. For studies, such as clinical trials, partnerships between communities and academic institutions have facilitated a greater diversity of subjects. Here, the benefit to the community is the development of standards of care that incorporate the social belief structure and needs of diverse communities.

The resources necessary to conduct quality research within community health centers are also being defined. The complexity of establishing research programs within health centers is astounding. Health centers operate on a very tight budget with little room for new programs and development. Therefore, major efforts to this date have focused on developing the infrastructure required to implement research and identifying funding sources to support such activities.

Committee on Government Affairs

The last two committees, Government Affairs and Finance, have interrelated responsibilities. The Government Affairs Committee is responsible for defining the policy agenda of CCHERS. It also delineates strategies for informing policymakers of legislation and regulation as they pertain to the mission of CCHERS.

Finance Committee

The Finance Committee is charged with oversight of the budget planning and implementation and devising methods for the financial sustainability of CCHERS. Policy and sustainability are linked, and the two committees have cross-representation and shared staff support.

Administrative Staff

The administrative staff of CCHERS provides the overall leadership and direction of the projects delegated by the board of directors (see Figure 1.3). The executive director reports to the board through the Executive Committee. All administrative and support staff of the project report to the executive director. The staff is composed of the executive director, project evaluator, policy an-

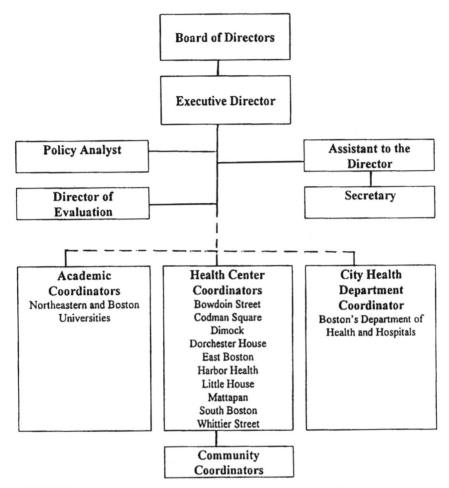

FIGURE 1.3 Administrative structure, Center for Community Health Education, Research, and Service.

alyst, media specialist, development officer, and administrative support staff, for a total of six full-time equivalent positions fully funded through the Kellogg Foundation grant.

Institution-Based Staff

The rest of the staff of the project is located within the various institutions of the partnership with an indirect, though strong reporting link to the executive director. Staff members are responsible for implementing the project within a particular site in collaboration with the other partner institutions. These institution-based personnel are responsible for implementing the policies of the board of directors, as guided by the executive director, in a manner congruent with the needs and values of the individual agency. This category of personnel reports directly to the respective administrator in either the academic or community setting. The nature of this project requires strong communication networks between the partners. The coordinators serve as a vital link in this process.

Coordination

There is a coordinator for CCHERS for both the College of Nursing and the School of Medicine. The university coordinators provide the leadership within the academic setting to incorporate the philosophy and policies of CCHERS into curriculum planning. University coordinators work closely with the faculty to identify the students' learning needs. They then collaborate directly with their counterpart in the neighborhood health center to determine learning opportunities that encompass educational and community needs.

The staff for the project at each of the neighborhood health centers is composed of a coordinator for health professions education and a community coordinator. The former works directly with the academic institution's coordinators in planning student experiences. The schedule for each class of students is developed, along with the learning goals and the nature of the learning experiences the faculty is seeking. The neighborhood health center coordinator works with the staff at the neighborhood health center, as well as with adjacent and cooperating community affiliates (e.g. senior citizens day programs, school system, VNA, etc.) to explore possibilities for student learning. The community coordinator, much like a community outreach worker, endeavors through his or her contacts with the residents of the community to facilitate student involvement in the richness of the community's learning opportunities.

The coordinators fill a critical role in the identification and development of clinical learning opportunities. In the neighborhood health center, coordinators know the services offered on-site and those in the surrounding neighborhood. Initially, students' learning experiences in the community-based project were to be restricted to the neighborhood health centers. It rapidly became apparent, however, that outreach to agencies within the catchment area of the neighborhood health center would greatly enhance the students' learning opportunities, in terms of the nature and diversity of the experiences but, more important, in helping the student become part of the community. Outreach across the community has greatly expanded student perception of the lives of the residents, promoting depth in understanding, and approaching needs in a holistic manner.

Over the course of the project strong and productive collaborative relationships have developed between the "team" at each neighborhood health center (the coordinator, College of Nursing faculty, and participating agency physicians and nurses). Although continuity of all personnel has not been possible, a strong effort has been made to retain the same faculty members at each site. As the student complement has increased every year and each successive year of students is incorporated, additional faculty members have been added.

University Faculty

Faculty members from the universities are essential participants in CCHERS although they are not supported by Kellogg Foundation funds. In the model of nursing education, faculty members are on site with students for a clinical experience. Leaders in the College of Nursing specifically did not want to finance faculty positions from "soft" funds. Rather, the dean believed it was essential to build into the project the long-term commitment of direct faculty support, clearly establishing that community-based primary care experiences were integral components of the curriculum. This approach has required a shifting of college funds from faculty members teaching in hospital settings to support of the education occurring within communities. This strategy has provided for the total integration of the community-based education by moving this approach to the core of the College of Nursing's educational model.

Medicine uses a different approach to education. In the medical model, clinical education is provided by faculty members at the clinical site, whether attending physicians in a hospital setting or primary care physicians in a health center. These clinical faculty members are adjunct faculty of the School of Medicine and work in close collaboration with the university coordinator to design the learning experiences for students. As with the College of Nursing, no direct funding from CCHERS is provided for the university-based medical faculty.

The faculty members located within the community health center work closely with the coordinators of health professions education, the community coordinators, the staff of the health center, and community residents. Each of these individuals is part of the extended faculty through the CCHERS model, and many have adjunct appointments with the College of Nursing. Financial support has been provided to the community health centers to develop a cadre of faculty to support the education of both nursing and medical students. This funding offsets some of the cost of staff time diverted from normal responsibilities of patient care to student education. The most significant financial impact of education with the health centers is a potential loss of revenue if providers see fewer clients while precepting students. For a quality educational experience, nurses, doctors, social workers, and others must have additional time to review approaches, assessments, diseases, treatments, patient responses, and other aspects of care. As students mature in their professional capabilities and provide direct care, the health center receives professional assistance from them.

In addition to the time health center staff and community members spend working directly with students, they participate in faculty development and preparing for student experiences. This takes time, time that would have generated revenue through patient visits. Therefore, CCHERS has allocated funding to cushion this reduction of revenue, and long-term financial support for this change of work allocation within the health center is being sought through policy initiatives.

Consistent with requirements of various standards for higher education and the professions, community-based staff assist the university faculty to develop bases in the community and identify experiences with the potential of fostering student learning. Thus, the community partnership is operationalized on many levels: at the grass roots between students, faculty members, and residents of the community; between program planners, administrators, and community boards; between faculty administrators and clinical staff of the neighborhood health center; and within the leadership of each partner organization.

Over the course of the project the knowledge base among the participants, faculty, and students has evolved with regard to all aspects of the project. There was a gradual learning about the role of the community and the way in which various agencies could participate as sites for students' experiences. Over time faculty members have begun to view the neighborhood health center as the hub of community-based services with multiple spokes reaching out across the neighborhood.

Outcome of Implementation

As with all efforts to help groups with differing priorities and frames of reference form bonds, the implementation of all aspects of the partnership has been very time consuming, requiring extensive dialogue and negotiation. The development of a clinical network to provide meaningful and appropriate learning experiences for the students requires ongoing discussion and assessment. The CCHERS partnership has taught participants much about the possibilities of a redefinition of colleagues working together in new coalitions. All partners in the consortium may have similar long-range goals and ideals, but they are, by the nature of their organizations and missions, disparate. The need to listen closely and to hear the messages of other partners became evident early in the development of the consortium. Although they used the same words members of the communities, universities, and health care agencies understood them differently. A partnership is a sharing process; consequently, it is essential that it be based on trust and a genuine belief that each partner has a concern and a commitment to every other partner.

CHALLENGES AND ACCOMPLISHMENTS

The development and implementation of community-based primary care in this college of nursing has been difficult. Change is always a challenge. Radical change, such as that occurring in the health care system, jeopardizes the security of known approaches. Further, the degree to which individuals are able to see that the change in the broadened system requires a personal change varies. The magnitude of this project in its fundamental attempt to redirect health professions education is basically threatening to the traditions of nursing education. Coupled with the transformation of inpatient nursing services, nurse educators find themselves in an intimidating circumstance. Despite the changing health care environment, perceptions of the need for educational change vary significantly among faculty. The magnitude of the actual change is fiercely debated, with some faculty members resisting redirection. Reasons vary. Some simply expect the health care system alterations to be minimal; others fear loss of their vested interests as changes leave them unprepared for new systems.

Teaching in the health centers and communities is difficult. All participants are teaching in a new approach or for the first time; hence, their skills also vary. Providers and other community-based faculty members are new to teaching, and their skills also vary. Many teach as they were taught, with differing results. Consequently, there is less capability to anticipate students' needs and responses. All the project and neighborhood health center staff participating in the education of students require development, support, and guidance from each other and acknowledgment from the formal system. The university faculty members are also uncertain about how to teach in the new environment. Teaching methodologies effective in the institutional setting do not capture the richness of the community experience. New approaches must be discovered. The result is shared learning and recognition of different expertise.

Multidisciplinary education is a philosophical struggle and very time-consuming. Reaching consensus on what should be taught, who should teach it, and when it should be taught is not easy. The understanding of each other's profession is limited among the collective faculty, and many misunderstandings exist. Faculty members need to clarify the areas of shared knowledge and skills among disciplines before this information can be presented to students. Multidisciplinary orientations are further clouded as each individual profession attempts to identify the essential knowledge required for community-based primary care education. Therefore, essential curriculum concepts are being defined at many levels, including those specific to a discipline (such as nursing), those required for responsive community care, and those shared across disciplines, forming the basis for multidisciplinary experiences.

Moreover, complicating the multidisciplinary approach is the reality that multidisciplinary teams in practice are more often the exception than the rule. How do you teach and model something that is just developing in practice? Achieving success demands committed believers in multidisciplinary care and education and the honesty to share evaluative information, thoughts, and goals openly.

The difference in focus between a health center and a university presents an important lesson. Universities have a primary mission to educate students. Community health centers have a primary mission to provide health services. Although there is considerable overlap in activities, it takes work to bring the two together. Similarly, community involvement in academic processes creates a clash of cultures. Universities are conceptual, idealistic, and traditional. Communities (health centers) are pragmatic, realistic, and contemporary. As the two cultures converge there are struggles with power, control, and respect. This is not unlike the struggles over education and service that universities and hospitals experience. The major difference, however, is the nature of the community. It does not have a defined organizational structure with clear paths of entry and mechanisms for negotiation. Communities are diffuse with multiple leaders, many factions, and long histories. The development of trust within communities cannot be rushed but needs opportunities to be tested and challenged. When providers care for a person from another culture, they must clearly understand their own value system and its influence in their interactions. Likewise, they must learn the value system of the other person to understand his/her approach to the interaction. This takes time and a great deal of give-and-take.

Moving research to the community meets with similar challenges. Community-based research is often not valued by academicians, whereas traditional research is not valued by communities. Neither meets the other's needs. A modification, a blend is necessary. Adding to the challenge are limited sources of funding for community-based research and a limited pool of seasoned researchers ready to change direction to a new methodology in the community. Many false starts can be expected as the process moves forward.

Acknowledging the ever-present challenges, many successes have been achieved. Health professions students' attitudes are changing; new systems of care are being developed; and existing agencies are joining the process of educating student. Many examples of successes in the educational change are presented in the following chapters.

Health centers are seeing successes as well. Recruitment and retention of all ranges of providers and staff are improving. Roles of teacher and researcher augment providers' practice responsibilities, and they express greater satisfaction with their work. New staff members are easier to recruit. Despite the obstacles identified, the academic community health care systems are forming through the partnerships of universities and communities. A common vision and interinstitutional trust continues to grow.

SUMMARY

Through the collaboration of a consortium of hospital, medical school, nursing college, and community health centers, students are being prepared to practice in the system evolving through health care reform. The most important outcome of the described model of education is the preparation of nurses and doctors for a new health care delivery system.

In 1995 the CCHERS project completed its fourth year of actual operation. During the development and implementation of the academic-community partnership, issues of power and control, protection of turf, competition among partners, and the challenges of sustainability have all arisen. The issues remain although there is a concurrent growth of trust and a long-standing working relationship that greatly facilitate collaboration. Initially, the consortium was viewed as a peripheral project for all of the organizations. It was an opportunity to provide diverse learning experiences for students. Over the past 4 years, however, the pressure on academic institutions to produce primary care practitioners has increased, and community health centers have been forced to examine their role in educating future providers.

The magnitude of the external pressures creates new tensions within the consortium. As the partnership becomes more important to the central role of each organization, the power of the consortium threatens each individual organization. The negotiated roles and turf lines have been blurred, and new tensions have evolved in the continuous push-pull nature of this alliance. Most evident in this process is the move toward further development of graduate education programs and the sharing of long-term funding.

Much has been gained from this partnership. The member organizations value its existence and future direction. The student learning experiences have been multidisciplinary in both student mix and faculty representation. Traditional nursing and medical education have been enriched with opportunities to integrate community, social, and public health issues into primary care. The diversity of community groups allows students to gain an in-depth knowledge of many cultures and many different living styles. From each interaction they learn about the challenges and successes of community residents. Equally important, they learn how to use their medical or nursing knowledge outside the hospital or health center walls.

Benefits to the member organizations reflect the focus of each institutional mission. Community health centers are realizing an increased ability to recruit and retain providers. Morale is enhanced, and services are expanded as students reach the later stages of their respective academic programs. The universities have the opportunity to expose students to a model of comprehensive, community-based primary care in the inner-city environment. Although communities provide the learning experience, they also gain, with increased services through the academic-community linkage. Finally, the hospital has the advantage of an improved referral network for patients through growing collaborations with community health center providers.

As the health care reform train leaves the station and builds up speed, educators must be sure they are on board. Many curricula offered to students are outdated. The flood of new information is so great, faculty members cannot pretend to teach all that needs to be known. Rather, the challenge to educators is to teach a thought process, critical thinking, and to socialize students to multiple environments where their talents are useful.

Reforms must include support to change both the delivery and educational systems that will provide the future work force. Collective partnerships of university, service agencies, and communities must inform policymakers of the blend of resources needed for a successful transformation.

REFERENCES

Bowman, R. A. (1992). Nursing returns to the home health frontier: Markets and trends in home health care. In L. Aiken & C. Fagin (Eds.), *Charting nursing's future agenda for the 1990's* (pp. 235–254). Philadelphia: Lippincott.

Boyer, E. L. (1991). *Scholarship reconsidered: Priorities of the professorate.* Princeton, NJ: The Carnegie Foundation.

Community partnerships: Redirecting health professions education toward primary care. (1992). Battle Creek, MI: W. K. Kellogg Foundation.

Lake, E. (1992). Medicare prospective payment and the changing health care environment. In L. Aiken & C. Fagin (Eds.), *Charting nursing's future agenda for the 1990's* (pp. 121–138). Philadelphia: Lippincott.

Massachusetts Rate Setting Commission. (1994). *Preventable hospitalization in Massachusetts.* Boston: Commonwealth of Massachusetts.

National Association of Community Health Centers. (1993). *Access to community health care: a national and state data book.* Washington, DC: Author.

National League for Nursing. (1993). *A vision for nursing education.* New York: Author.

Pew Health Professions Commission. (1991). *Health American: Practitioners for 2005. An agenda for action for health professions schools.* Durham, NC: Pew Foundation.

Shields, J., & Wolfe, P. (1992). *The role of private health insurance.* Washington, DC: Lewwin-ICF.

Wofford, H. (1980). *Of Kennedy and kings.* Pittsburgh, PA: University of Pittsburgh Press.

Young, D. (1982). *A promise kept: Boston's neighborhood health centers.* Boston: Trustees of Health and Hospitals.

2

Laying the Groundwork for Curriculum Change

Carole A. Shea

Schools of nursing are feeling pressure from several quarters to transform nursing education. National efforts to reform health care are one obvious source. More subtle but just as pervasive is the public's criticism of institutions of higher learning (Bok, 1992). Although the criticism has not been directed at nursing curricula per se, the public's suspicion that academe cannot be trusted to educate students in a cost-effective manner for the rapidly changing world of tomorrow could potentially affect support for nursing programs.

PRESSURES TO REFORM ACADEME

The public expects its institutions of higher education to prepare students to earn a living; expand the liberal arts and sciences by stimulating learning and critical thinking, and make a contribution to the advancement of a democratic society (Stimpson, 1992). Efforts to meet these expectations in general education have led to considerable debate, both inside and outside academe, about such issues as cultural diversity, the relevance of scholarly studies to the reality of the workplace, faculty workload, and scientific integrity.

Ultimately, the public is most concerned about its return on investment, in terms of cost, pricing, access, productivity, outcomes, and effectiveness of higher education. These concerns are manifested in many ways. There is the basic anxiety about how a single individual, the family, or tax-paying citizens of a community can afford to send a student to college as tuition costs continue to soar. There is puzzlement about the basic mission of the university: is it primarily to teach students or to conduct research? There is heated controversy over curriculum, not just its content but also its goals and methods of achieving them. There is outrage over the scandalous behavior of fraudulent researchers and greedy administrators at leading universities. There is dissatisfaction with institutions' ability to come to grips with a changing world—its economy, technology, demography, and globalization—and to provide a blueprint for the future.

Nursing is not immune to the pressures created by these criticisms despite its long-standing commitment to serving society's needs; attention to the rigors of curriculum development, evaluation, and accreditation; and adherence to an established code of professional ethics. Members of nursing school faculties are participants in the discourse about the role of academe in society and competitors for the financing of public life. They must become more actively engaged in redefining the university's mission, transforming curricula, assuring the quality of educational programs, and regaining trust through ethical behavior to justify the cost of nursing education to society.

We are in the midst of a health care delivery revolution, yet nursing educators are only beginning to come to grips with a curriculum that will meet the demands of the workplace and serve the needs of society in the coming century. However, spurred on by the profession's vision (ANA, 1991; NLN, 1993), a number of nursing faculties are on the move to provide educational tools for the next generation of nurses and retool for opportunities for those who are committed to improving practice.

EXPECTATIONS OF NURSING EDUCATION

Nursing education has not become embroiled in the controversies surrounding general higher education because, so far, its programs have met the public's expectations. Degree-granting programs have produced competent professional nurses, expanded the art and science of nursing, and contributed to society by improving the health of its citizens. Before resting on laurels, however, faculty members must reexamine nursing programs in light of the recent trends in education and health care. Broadly speaking, both education and health care reform are concerned with access, quality, and cost-effectiveness. These factors have a major impact on the learning process, the nursing curriculum, and the clinical learning opportunities for nursing students.

The Learning Process

The learning process, more accurately termed the "teaching-learning process," is the heart of the educational enterprise. Key values influence who teaches and who learns, as well as how the teaching and learning take place. Some of the most influential values and principles in nursing education today are related to diversity, shared human experience, autonomy, conceptualization, and lifelong learning. These are in stark contrast to the values and principles that guided nursing education in the past, such as conformity, procedure-based experience, supervision, tradition, and rote learning.

The valuing of diversity means that differences (e.g., age, gender, race, culture, and sexual orientation) among nursing students, as well as patient populations, are recognized, appreciated, and taken into consideration. For example, faculty members give more than lip service to principles of adult learning when they empower students to design different study methods for learning about health assessment skills. Some students may choose to practice skills with a peer partner in the nursing laboratory; some may prefer extensive review using simulated or self-paced learning modules in the library; some may require supervised practice sessions with the instructor on a clinical unit. The defining principles are that (1) there is no one right way to learn, and (2) adult students who are self-directed know best how they learn.

Given the increasing diversity of students entering the nursing profession—more men, older students, more career changers, more ethnic diversity in the student body—more ways to learn, greater use of technology (and teaching of ways to use technology appropriately), more flexibility in scheduling learning experiences, greater variety in learning experiences, and more creative ways to evaluate how and when learning takes place are needed.

Increased diversity places a premium on the faculty member who is innovative, tolerant of ambiguity, and sensitive to the individual learning needs and teaching potential of each nursing student.

The shift to valuing the shared human experience is an outcome of the phenomenon of caring in nursing practice. Educators are recognizing that students cannot learn to "care," or to "provide care," by concentrating on practice with manikins in a laboratory or following procedural guides that ignore human variation and the healing power of interpersonal exchange. Therefore, the faculty must focus the teaching-learning process on caring with and for people who are in the throes of experiencing health and illness within the context of their daily lives. Students must be taught to embrace professional ethics but not to use "professionalism" as a rationale to distance themselves from involvement with their patients or to objectify the nurse-patient relationship. Learning, teaching, and decision making are shared experiences in the student-patient interaction.

Autonomy, with its intimation of self-governance, self-direction, and independence, has long been a hallmark of the professions. In nursing, autonomy is a reality sometimes, but more often it is a wished for quality. In part, nurses' struggle for autonomy may be related to many nursing faculties' assumption that autonomy cannot be taught or learned prior to graduation and licensure as a registered nurse. The legacy of strict, ever-present supervision of nursing students and novice nurses communicates a lack of confidence in their ability to exercise good judgment and be accountable for their behavior. The expectation that autonomy is unwarranted (and unwanted) prior to achieving expert status prevents nurses, and certainly students, from exercising autonomy that is appropriate to their stage of professional development. Autonomy is not a zero-sum concept; there are levels of autonomy. Forward-thinking educators know that autonomy, like trust, develops over time when situations of graduated complexity are presented to the learner, together with the requisite background of knowledge, skills, and professional support.

Conceptualization, or the teaching of information by providing meaning through the explication of conceptual relationships, rather than a laundry list of facts, is not new to nursing. In their heyday, nursing theorists proposed concepts, frameworks, models, and theories to define, explain, and synthesize the knowledge, skills, and attitudes that comprise the discipline of nursing. Over time, nursing theories have not lived up to their promise. The context of nursing practice has become too complex, too varied, and too specialized to subscribe to one theoretical model.

Today, the emphasis must be on how to learn (process), not what to learn (content). There is simply too much information to try to pack it all into a standard professional nursing program. Instead, faculty members are stressing critical thinking skills, information literacy, clinical decision making, outcome measurement, and interdisciplinary collaboration as the essential nursing tools for the next century.

Even with heuristic devices for learning, rather than lectures of discrete facts, nursing curricula are packed with content. The learning curve is steep as students and faculty grapple with basic sciences, social sciences, the humanities, and the art and science of nursing itself. Determining what is a priority and what is outdated or irrelevant for the future is a very difficult task. In the face of the Great Unknown of ever-changing health care, faculty face tough choices. For example, which disease entity or particular age group should they select as a prototype for learning effective nursing interventions? Should they include studies in economics or in genetics as required courses? Some solutions to these dilemmas are to rely more on the individual student's prior knowledge, experiences, preferences, and responsibility for her or his own learning; capitalize on the student peers' shared teaching-learning moments to a greater extent, rather than always structuring the learning opportunities as a faculty-student interaction; and inculcate the value of lifelong learning by professional socialization and personal example.

Lifelong learning is becoming a fact of life for all society. With the average person projected to have more than three careers in a life time, the presumption that students can learn all they need to know in one program or at one point in time is ludicrous. This is particularly true in a field such as nursing in which the science is still emerging and practice is evolving to a higher level of complexity. Educators who are comfortable in portraying the need to keep learning, not the need to "know all" will be modeling a valuable lesson to nursing students.

The Nursing Curriculum

Given the ongoing restructuring in health care and higher education and the changes in the teaching-learning process, profound
implications exist for the nursing curriculum of tomorrow. The
landmark Pew Health Professions Commission Report (1991) referred to in chapter 1 of this book, represents a convergence of
thinking about the need for curriculum revision in health professions education. The changes proposed in the Pew Report may
be summarized as follows:

- A major focus on health and primary health care delivery.
- Increased emphasis on health promotion and maintenance
  through teaching and counseling interventions.
- Inclusion of individuals, families, and communities in decisions affecting their health and treating their illnesses.
- A commitment to understanding, appreciating, and working
  with underserved populations.
- The need for an interdisciplinary approach and teamwork to
  deliver comprehensive care.
- A deeper understanding and appreciation of the role of the
  community in the health of individuals, families, and their
  community.

Most undergraduate nursing curricula are organized in some
way around a continuum of care ranging from health promotion
to providing care and comfort to the dying, with consideration of
individuals' health and illness issues throughout their life span.
Many programs have evolved sophisticated frameworks for guid-
ing students to provide care through the nursing process. Despite the use of nursing models and wellness rhetoric most nursing students spend the majority of their study time and clinical
learning experiences concentrating on disease processes and care
of sick individuals in hospitals. If the distinguishing feature of
nursing as a health profession is its expertise in health promotion, health maintenance, and health restoration, this feature
must be evident in lecture time and clinical assignments. To make
substantive changes in nursing education, as the Pew Report
suggests, the curriculum will have to change in several fundamental ways.

1. *Students must be socialized to regard health, not disease, as the paramount concern of nursing.* This would suggest that nursing courses should start with health as the primary topic, perhaps beginning with the health of the student as a consumer to increase its immediacy and relevance. Health teaching and health counseling should be promoted as very important functions of the nurse, not as "nice-to-do activities, if you have time."

2. *Primary care interventions to promote, maintain, and restore health must be taught based on the latest scientific research and state-of-the-art nursing practice.* These interventions are every bit as complex as those involving sophisticated technology and pharmacology. Epidemiological and behavioral sciences would have to be incorporated into the curriculum to provide the knowledge base for effective health interventions.

3. *Health problems and concerns must be reinforced throughout the curriculum, not just in introductory courses.* Pertinent health and wellness issues exist at every stage of illness. Health may be defined as the sense of well-being, a holistic and dynamic force that occurs within the context of wellness and illness. Teaching levels of prevention must be an integral part of every course, with specific clinical examples provided. This would necessitate spending proportionately less class time on etiology of disease and more on nursing interventions along the continuum of well-being.

4. *Foundation and supporting courses must be chosen with an eye toward their relevance for delivery of nursing services that are health- as well as illness-oriented; consideration of the mission of the institution; and contribution to the science of nursing.* Because of constraints within the standard 4-year collegiate program, this will require faculty members to rethink credit allocation to nursing and non-nursing courses, make trade-offs between required basic and social science courses, and sacrifice elective credits in favor of required science, art, humanities, or nursing courses. Some programs may be further constrained by state board of nursing requirements or the core curriculum demands of their institution. A thoughtful rationale with documentation for proposed changes may go a long way to smoothing the path to curriculum revision.

To make the substantive changes outlined in these four points, the nursing curricula must have an increased emphasis on community-based primary health care. The promotion of health across the life-span for individuals, families, groups, and communities must focus on the context in which people experience health and illness.

One way to organize the nursing curriculum is to present, in the first nursing course, the component of community-based primary care, with its emphasis on health promotion and disease prevention. This sets a frame of reference for all subsequent clinical courses. Throughout the program students learn the breadth and depth of knowledge, skills, contexts, perspectives, and attitudes they need to provide health care that is comprehensive, culturally sensitive, continuous, effective, compassionate, and collaborative. The knowledge and skills base for the community-based primary care component includes those traditionally associated with assessment, diagnosis, and treatment of illness. However, there is a greater emphasis on skills, such as comprehensive assessments of individuals, families, and communities; diagnosing health problems, as well as disease conditions; and using a broader array of intervention strategies, including shared decision making, conflict resolution, community planning, disease prevention, and epidemiological research. Such a curriculum is intended to provide a balance to the students learning about primary, secondary, and tertiary levels of care that is reflective of national health care goals for the improved health of the whole population.

CLINICAL LEARNING OPPORTUNITIES

The essence of any professional education lies in the way the students are taught to practice the discipline. In nursing, the majority of students' clinical instruction takes place in hospitals, large and small. These organizations are characterized by structured authority lines, high technology, and episodic care of patients with acute medical-surgical illnesses.

The few out-of-hospital clinical experiences generally come at the culmination of the program, when students have already become thoroughly socialized to high-tech, bureaucratic medicine. In theory, the community health practicum, usually through a Visiting Nurses Association (VNA) affiliation, is an opportunity for students to synthesize all they have learned (in the hospital setting) while caring for a convalescing or chronically ill person in a home setting. Without the usual supervision, professional backup, and equipment of the hospital, students are expected to get a taste of autonomous practice and learn how to deal with families on their own turf. For some students the community experience is a welcome breath of fresh air; for others it is a terrifying example of professional abandonment. At best, it is too little, too late in the socialization process to make a difference in how the students will practice in the future.

With the delivery of most health care moving out of the hospital to community settings, the focus of nursing curricula must shift its direction to respond to society's need for health care. Because the vast majority of people's lives are spent in their community, outside medical centers and hospitals, a significant and meaningful part of the education of nurses must take place in the community where people live, raise families, work, eat, rest, play, vote, and pray. This approach is concerned with the who, what, when, where, how, and why questions surrounding the health care of individuals, families, groups, and communities. For example, nurses seek to know and understand who people are in the fullest sense, where they live and with whom, what they do to sustain their way of life, how they play and have fun, what they contribute to a diverse society. In addition they learn where and why they seek health care and how they maintain their health, manage health problems, and respond to illness and treatment.

Clinical experiences that augment a community-based primary care nursing curriculum provide opportunities for students to

- participate in the experience of health and illness of individuals and families within the real-life context of the community;
- encounter the diversity of people and communities in a natural setting;
- make clinical judgments informed by the "big picture"—the social, cultural, legal, political, ecological, and epidemiological factors that affect health, illness, and response to programs and interventions; and

- share responsibility with patients, providers, and community residents for decisions affecting the health of the community.

If nursing educators are to institute meaningful curriculum change, to transform health rhetoric into a nursing practice reality, they will have to provide new and different clinical learning opportunities for nursing students. Examples of innovative clinical experiences are woven throughout the following chapters of this book.

THE NATURAL ADVANTAGE OF COMMUNITY SETTINGS

Restructuring the nursing curriculum around primary health care and community settings often has particular advantages for students, faculty, and community residents.

The Ocean: A Metaphor for Community-Based Primary Care

The following analogy demonstrates the special nature of an educational program of community-based learning by comparing participant reactions to that of swimmers experiencing the ocean for the first time.

Once there was an educational program designed to teach many different students how to swim in the Ocean of Primary Health Care. This ocean was very bountiful, so many people wanted to learn how to swim in it. The students came from many places with a variety of experiences. However, most of them came from a part of the country where there was no ocean; they had a wide variety of expectations about swimming in it.

Some students had previous experience swimming in ponds and lakes. They expected the ocean to have well-contained banks, a consistent waterline, and predictable depth. They were very surprised to learn about the ocean's varied shoreline and the effects of constantly changing tides. They marveled at the size of the waves and the variation in temperature of the water. They liked the sandy bottom, which was quite different from their experience of silt-filled ponds and lakes. When they entered the ocean, they were thrilled with the added buoyancy of the salt water. At first the pull of the tidal currents frightened them; but then they learned to ride the waves. Gradually, they learned to take advantage of the ocean's power as they became strong swimmers. A few even learned to teach others to swim and ride the waves on surfboards.

Another group of students also knew how to swim. They expected the ocean to be like the pools in their hometown, only larger. Imagine their surprise when they reached the seashore to find the ocean stretching to the farthest horizon. And what was that smell! Salt air? Mmm, much better than the familiar chlorine smell of the pool back home. When they ventured out into the water, they too enjoyed the waves. They were impressed that there were no time-consuming pool-cleaning chores or costly fees for using the ocean. But they were bothered by the ocean; the water wasn't temperature-controlled, and it wasn't crystal clear either. When they came out, they had to deal with sticky sand and salt . They became very doubtful that swimming in the ocean was such a good idea. They much preferred the artificial pool back home, where they could control the temperature, see the bottom at all times, and come out feeling clean, despite the whiff of pool disinfectant. They did think the ocean a good place for certain water sports, however. So from time to time, they spent a day whizzing around on a Jet Ski or crashing through the waves in a sleek powerboat. They were unconcerned about the oil slick they left on the water or the danger they might pose to people or fish swimming in their path or swamped by their wake.

Only a few students didn't know how to swim and had never been in a large body of water before. Of course, they had seen pools and lakes and swimmers on television and in movies, but they had no personal experience with swimming or swimmers. They didn't know quite what to expect. They were captivated by the natural beauty of the ocean—the sights, sounds, smells of the sea, the feel of ocean breezes, the interaction of sun, sand, wind, and water. They were amazed that the ocean seemed to have a way (a mind?) of its own; certainly, no one person could control it. But the ocean was so refreshing. In fact, it seemed to clean itself, washing things out to sea and returning treasures from the bottom for the collectors of shells, seaglass, and driftwood, as well as food for the shorebirds and other sea creatures.

At first it was frightening to try to learn to swim when the waves tossed them about, and they couldn't see exactly where they were going. Fortunately, they didn't have to plunge in, like those who had to dive headfirst into pools when they were learning to swim. Instead, these students could wade in slowly, take their time, feel their way, step carefully among the stones and shells. And jumping into the waves was fun. There was much less need to pay attention to swimmer's strokes and form; they could concentrate on the pleasure of the moment. There always seemed to be plenty of people around who knew what to do and were happy to show them the water tricks they knew. The sticky sand and salt didn't bother these students as much because they accepted it as a natural part of the ocean. Gradually, they began to feel very comfortable in the ocean, to respect its power and enjoy its bounty. In time, they learned to swim with those who spend their life improving their strokes and getting to know the ocean better.

The community as the Ocean of Primary Health Care, is a powerful natural entity that commands strong feelings, requires special skills, and offers an almost boundless opportunity for education, research, and service. It is not a "system"; it is messy, it is colorful, it is very real. Nurses and other health professionals develop preferences for "swimming in the ocean" (community-based primary care) or "in the pool" (hospital-based tertiary care). Students need ample guided experiences in both to understand the complexities of health care before they make an initial choice to practice in one or the other.

Nursing students' preferences are determined by the expectations they bring with them to their formal education, the nursing curriculum, their first clinical encounters, the behaviors of significant role models, the influence of peers, friends, and family, and so much more. Nursing education has been solidly entrenched in tertiary care. However, today's students need an early and prolonged exposure to the community "ocean experience" to prepare them for a rapidly transforming health care future. Shifting the weight of learning toward community-based primary care helps to prepare all nursing students to undertake the work of providing health care in whatever setting they may choose to practice.

Advantages for Students

In the community, nursing students may experience the full continuum of care and what it really means to provide continuity. When students are assigned to follow families, they may have the opportunity to witness firsthand the onset of illness, its treatment, and the restoration of health. Unlike nurses who work in critical care units, students in the community have a much more optimistic (and realistic) picture of what recovery means to the patient and family. In the community they see that patients return from the hospital and get well or learn to live with their chronic illness. Recovery models of nursing care should predominate, therefore, because "worst-case scenarios" are not usual in the community.

On the other hand, the issue of compliance takes on a whole new meaning when the individual and his or her family is in charge. Students confront the reality of medications that are too expensive to take as ordered or regimens that are too complicated to follow without educational materials translated into a specific language and dialect. Many times this is an opportunity for the family to teach the student about viable alternatives to the prescribed regimen. Sometimes, these family-devised interventions can be used again or modified to fit the needs of similar families.

Students learn that interventions tailored to meet the needs of the situation are often more effective because they are based on respect for the family's knowledge, sensitive to cultural beliefs and practices, and considerate of a family's resources. Over time, students gather evidence of the effectiveness of their interventions, learning what works and what does not, and why.

Immersion in an underserved urban or rural community setting promotes changes in attitudes as students become more comfortable with differences in race, culture, life-style, and economic class. This takes time, as the unfamiliar sights, sounds, smells, and environmental conditions of a neighborhood impinge on their predominantly white, middle-class sensitivities. But an understanding of the joys and difficulties of diverse groups of people can be empathy-building and personally enriching for students, especially those who lack prior experience with multicultural influences.

Learning opportunities in the community enrich the nurse-patient relationship in several ways. Nursing students learn to relate to more than one patient at a time, because most encounters are with more than just the primary client. They learn to communicate in a give-and-take manner, capitalizing on the therapeutic values of openness, authenticity, and empathy within the established relationship. They have a chance to practice multiple roles: that of direct caregiver, teacher, counselor, advocate, and case manager. They also extend the scope of practice by becoming involved in community projects, health fairs, after-school programs, surveys, and research.

Finally, nursing students learn the value of teamwork and collaboration with peers, providers, and community residents when they return to the same neighborhood and the community health center for ongoing learning experiences. Teams take time to build. Community health centers, by virtue of their size and philosophy, provide a living laboratory of how health professionals can work together as partners with community residents. In many cases this is only an ideal, but the elements are there for students and faculty to develop into a workable model.

Advantages for Faculty

The advantages of a community practice setting for faculty are those of a vast, untapped resource. Whereas nurses have always practiced in the community using public health or VNA models, community health practice today requires a new model. The clientele, the clinical problems, the reimbursement system, the mind set of the consumer, even the professional providers have changed. The transformation of health care is dictating a new playing field, with new rules and new players.

Nursing practice in the community is fertile ground for testing new ideas and creating new roles. For example, nurse practitioners are well established in community health centers, but the role of the baccalaureate-prepared nurse is not. Faculty members have an unique opportunity to introduce the nurse with a baccalaureate degree, who has a broad array of knowledge and skills, into a setting where many of the desired health services cannot be offered because busy practitioners must concentrate on delivering direct care. The range of activities in which the baccalaureate student might engage is almost limitless. Faculty members can then witness and evaluate the effectiveness of the nurse educated in a program that stresses primary health care and community-based values.

In the community, nursing educators have new avenues for carrying out research and exploring other professional interests. For example, the field for studying health promotion strategies is wide open. Although community members are not eager to become research "guinea pigs," research methods that involve residents in the definition of the problem, as well as the interventions and solutions, may be welcomed and fill a serious void in community health and health services research. Research is also one of the best ways to forge collaborative partnerships with professional peers, students, and community residents. Frequently, seeking approval for research projects is much less cumbersome, although competition for subjects may still prove difficult.

Many community sites will provide options for faculty practice. Faculty members may wish to practice as part of their workload, to demonstrate a positive role model for students, maintain their advanced certification, or provide a service to the community. Arrangements can be structured that benefit the agency, as well as to update or keep faculty members current in their specialty. Some schools of nursing now require faculty members teaching clinical courses to demonstrate their clinical expertise or participate in the school's faculty practice plan. Often, there is considerably more flexibility in scheduling practice sessions within a community health center or other community-based agency than in hospitals. Further, as hospitals downsize, fewer openings for part-time work or per diem shifts for faculty are available. Practice in the community may be an attractive alternative.

For those faculty accustomed to working only in hospitals, the move to the community may represent quite a challenge. But challenges sometimes present themselves as a stimulus for change. Faculty members may well be energized by the need to develop new content areas and creative teaching methodologies to fit nursing practice in the community. The trend toward the "graying of the faculty" means that many nursing faculty members have been teaching at the same institution, in the same courses, with the same clinical affiliations for several years. They may welcome the disruption in all that sameness, as they seek new information, find new colleagues, and use new resources to teach a broader scope of nursing to new students.

Advantages for the Community

The community stands to benefit, too, as faculty and students try to bring the academic perspective to health care in the community. An increased access to expanded health services and programs is anticipated because of the combined effect of more funding for health professions education in the community and more reimbursement for services delivered in community-based settings.

A concomitant benefit may be derived from the increase in relevant research that tends to accompany faculty practice and active student clinical teaching. This would include not only the generation of more research but also the better use and dissemination of research findings. However, to truly benefit the community, its residents must be involved throughout the research process. Several research methods foster involvement, such as action research, ethnography, and community needs assessments. Other research projects, including the more traditional experimental designs, may be permitted as long as the community gives its approval and informed consent.

Community residents may also become actively involved in the education of future nurses and other health professionals, helping to create providers who are compassionate, culturally competent, socially responsible, and politically aware, as well as clinically proficient. This requires a teaching-learning process that is a two-way street between patient and provider. It also means that faculty and students must recognize community residents, in a variety of roles, as having the capacity to teach valuable information that has a bearing on health practices and outcomes. For example, the local clergy, police officer, bus driver, a grandmother, or a teenage basketball player all have the potential to make an important contribution to the education of nursing students.

The presence of students and their interactions with community residents at close quarters may also help recruit residents into health professions. Serving as appropriate role models and mentors, students and faculty may be able to break down the barriers that have prevented people indigenous to the community from becoming health providers. In this and other ways the community can become empowered to improve its health status and quality of life.

BARRIERS TO MOVING TO THE COMMUNITY

With all the advantages inherent in the community-based practice of nursing, it might seem as if the decision to move the curriculum from its traditional base would be relatively easy. But even a desired change is difficult to initiate and then implement. Despite the many positive forces for change, human nature resists. Barriers such as student reluctance, faculty resentment, and community skepticism often impede progress.

Student Reluctance

Students have difficulty moving to the community because of their traditional image of what nursing is and what nurses do. In part this is a reflection of public media presentations. With few exceptions, movies and television still portray nurses as women in starched white (some times with caps) who spend most of their time ministering to the patient's tubes and monitors or discussing personal matters with the doctor. Almost always, the nurse is located in a hospital, whereas in reality less than 65% are now employed in hospitals. Stories in the news describe the heroic measures of the critical care or emergency room nurses in life-and-death situations. So the majority of students who choose nursing expect to practice in a hospital, preferably on a fast-paced unit, at a relatively high starting salary. And they expect their clinical rotations to prepare them for that eventuality.

Their surprise and outright disappointment are all too evident when faculty members take them to a low-tech, slower-paced, small community center that provides health services for a non-captive group of residents, some of whom are unable to keep their appointments. The student's cognitive dissonance can be profound. Some will be intrigued, but many have great difficulty adjusting to the loss of their dream. Reworking the vision of what nursing is and will be in the future is a full-time occupation for the educators who attempt to teach community-based primary care to adult students with very different ideas.

Sometimes the difficulty for students is compounded by the unfamiliar territory they find themselves in and their fear of the unknown. Communities achieve their unique character by defining who is "in" and who is "out" as much as by geographic boundaries. Being on the "outs," a stranger, and having to prove oneself as worthy of acceptance by a dissimilar group is a confusing, uncomfortable experience for most individuals, including students and faculty. Having to learn a new role as one seeks acceptance is a definite challenge.

A particular problem in the community is the amount of time and investment of self required for a successful learning experience. With many nursing students working at least part-time in addition to their studies, time is a precious commodity. Community clinical experiences often require additional travel to and from more than one site within a neighborhood; they may require that the student take public transportation or have access to a car. Establishing relationships with community residents as well as designated clients is key—and takes time and personal initiative. Community health programs are not scheduled for the convenience of students and other providers. To interact with clients, students may be required to attend events in the evening or on weekends in addition to or instead of their regularly scheduled clinical time. Even the most enthusiastic and dedicated students may sometimes find it difficult to do all they wish to do within community-based primary health care.

For some students, the potential barriers are overcome once they acquire a new vision of nursing, learn how to move into the community, and figure out how to schedule their time. For others, their own stereotypes, prejudices. and other negative attitudes prove formidable and almost guarantee a difficult learning experience. Attitudes are hard to change, and the community becomes impatient with students and faculty members who project their negativity and insensitivity onto all around them. Special workshops on diversity, simulation games, one-to-one mentoring, peer advising, journal writing, and limit-setting on objectionable behavior all assist in dealing with students who continue to manifest biases toward the community learning experience.

Faculty members should anticipate that some students will exhibit reluctance to learn in the community setting and should structure their introduction to the neighborhood in a positive manner that allows for the welcoming by residents and providers. With exposure, information, support, and time, most students can make a valuable contribution to health care in the community and their own professional and personal growth. To promote a positive learning experience, faculty members should cultivate openness, caring, curiosity, and camaraderie among students. The most effective technique is for faculty members to model these characteristics in the interactions with patients, providers, and community residents.

Faculty Resentment

Faculty members respond to some of the same influences as do students. Their reluctance, however, may take the form of individual resentment or resistance to change.

Unlike the unsuspecting students, who are new to the nursing program, faculty members have had a long-established relationship with the traditional nursing curriculum. Moving longitudinal clinical experiences into the community gives rise to painful feelings associated with losing a curriculum that many view as their life's work. Moving toward community-based primary health care involves turning away from a curriculum that was carefully built, has demonstrated a track record of success, provides the faculty with a sense of specialty expertise and clinical competence, and fosters the establishment of strong collegial relationships in one particular affiliation.

Whatever enjoyment might be experienced from creating something new, it is balanced by the inevitable pressures of the lengthy, time-consuming, probably conflictual process of curriculum revision. Faculty members do not undertake the change of a whole curriculum lightly. Countless hours are spent on the development of philosophies, goals, objectives, and finely detailed course syllabi. This time commitment itself is cause enough for tremendous resentment.

There are few signposts to guide faculty in designing a revolutionary curriculum. The adventurous ones may adopt the approach of throwing caution to the winds, to plan as they go, and experiment with what works in the community clinical area. The more cautious ones will be worried about the lack of accepted models, the need to dot *i*'s and cross *t*'s before setting foot in the community. Both groups may fear the possibility of receiving a negative review from accrediting bodies. The faculty's varied personal styles and professional approaches may create havoc in the academic halls as the curriculum is forged. However, concerns may be tempered by the fact that so many systems, agencies, and accrediting organizations are themselves undergoing change. Faculties can anticipate that an innovative approach to curriculum will be rewarded ultimately.

Faculty members may also resent the need to retool, upgrade their clinical skills, or learn an entirely new role. Their dismay stems from different sources. Some faculty members have competing demands on their time—family obligations, ongoing research, long commutes to work. Some have not practiced for years, and they now have to accept the role of a beginning student in a new specialty. Many cannot accept that retooling for the future is a necessity. They persist in viewing it as extra work on an already overburdened schedule. The extent of their resistance may be influenced by their perception of the extent of choice in the matter, whether they receive release time or additional compensation, or how convenient it is to obtain the requisite education and practice experience.

In addition to resentment about the logistics of changing a curriculum and learning new clinical skills, some faculty members are philosophically opposed to some of the basic tenets of community-based primary care. They may object to the commitment to share authority and decision making with patients and community residents. They may be unwilling to allow students to act autonomously in any situation, especially during the early portions of the program. They may oppose the practice of allowing those who are not officially designated nursing faculty to teach students and supervise basic nursing functions in the community. Their objections come from their bedrock belief that nursing must be taught by nurses. They believe it is their prerogative and responsibility to teach and supervise all nursing students in all learning activities. The thought of delegating or sharing their responsibility with people who are not nurses or with students raises fears of loss of authority and even of charges of malpractice.

Faculty members who have philosophical differences about how to plan and implement a community-based curriculum present the greatest challenge to a successful curriculum change. As most theories of change suggest, involving faculty at every step of the way in making the curriculum revision and deciding how to retool helps to minimize resistance. Administrators and faculty leaders must be sensitive to the personal and professional needs of faculty over the course of this incredibly difficult period (which may stretch over years). It helps to cultivate the following characteristics in faculty: flexibility and improvisation; tolerance of ambiguity; willingness to collaborate; and above all humor. Fortunately, most faculty members can activate some of these characteristics in themselves and others given a conducive environment and attention to their own sense of well-being over the long haul. Faculty retreats, recognition and award ceremonies, training sessions, and celebrations of milestones contribute to faculty cohesion and achievement of academic goals.

Community Skepticism

Barriers to acceptance of the new nursing curriculum by the community may be characterized as skepticism or cynicism among community leaders and residents. Those with a keen sense of history may remember the legions of "do-gooders"—outsiders who started programs, usually with public funds or grants, and then disappeared when the money ran out. Raising expectations and promoting false hopes for services did more harm to the community in the long run. Today a grant-funded program must have a plan to become self-sustaining, but many still fall short of this goal, leaving communities in the lurch.

Communities also resent the intrusion of insensitive strangers. They will no longer tolerate the condescending attitudes and unconscious prejudices of seemingly well-intentioned health professionals. Communication is blocked when community members cannot understand or appreciate the socialization and culture of the professional provider and the provider is oblivious to the culture and ethos of the community. Open discussion of mutual misunderstandings and distrust may broach the impasse. However, professionals must realize that the community has the weight of justice on its side. In underserved areas the social injustices endured by its residents have left a bitter legacy. Professionals must overcome the community's skepticism about their motives and methods by including the community as a partner in all phases of the educational program—planning, implementation, and evaluation. Once again, the mutuality of the teaching-learning process is paramount.

Forming a partnership with the community does not eliminate all difficulties. For many the notion of a true partnership with professionals is a new experience. As such, it takes time to acquaint community participants with their roles as major players, as well as the requirements and methods of curriculum development and implementation. The goals of a community-based primary care curriculum may be understood in a different way by the community or rejected altogether in favor of a more traditional high-tech medical approach. The community also is influenced by the media, which promotes disease-oriented medicine. Health promotion strategies and health maintenance programs may be difficult to sell when community members have had to contend with untreated illnesses and out-of-control chronic conditions for years. Their skepticism about the value of a health-oriented program is best challenged by effective interventions that link community concerns with positive health outcomes, such as screening programs for diabetes, hypertension, and tuberculosis, acquired immune deficiency syndrome (AIDS) education for middle-schoolers, and influenza immunization for the elderly.

Finally, the community must deal with the disruption in their normal routines, customs, and established relationships. New programs and new people with new ideas challenge the comfort level and convenience of the usual way of doing business. To the extent that routines, habits, and customs can be incorporated into the new programs, they are likely to be accepted more quickly. Using some of the techniques of the ethnographer can be helpful here. For example, faculty can act as participant-observers; students can question the community residents as key informers; and providers can combine folk practices with modern interventions to enhance treatment. In working with community partners, the faculty may stress that everyone needs to tolerate the long learning curve, that positive and negative input and feedback from the residents are expected and welcomed, and that the common goal is improved health for the community. At all times, faculty and students must remember that they are guests in the community until the community informs them otherwise.

SUMMARY

This chapter has discussed the need for education reform in nursing; the effects of a community-based primary health care approach to nursing education on the learning process, the nursing curriculum, and clinical learning opportunities; the advantages of community-based nursing education for students, faculty, and the community; and barriers to implementing such a program in the community. An analogy of the community as a natural entity for nursing education was also presented.

Although the challenge to make a location change in nursing education is formidable, the rewards are just as promising. Nursing educators have the external driving forces of education and health care reform and the internal visionary leadership to transform nursing education and practice before the end of this century. With stamina, courage, caring, and creativity they are meeting the challenge and enjoying the satisfaction and educational rewards that come with hard work and a commitment to service in a rapidly changing society.

REFERENCES

American Nurses Association. (1991). *Nursing's agenda for health care reform.* Washington, DC: Author.

Bok, D. (1992). Reclaiming the public trust. *Change, 24*(4) 12–19.

National League for Nursing. (1993). *A vision for nursing education.* New York: Author.

Pew Health Professions Commission. (1991). *Health American: Practitioners for 2005. An agenda for action for health professions schools.* Durham, NC: Author.

Stimpson, C. R. (1992). Some comments on curriculum: Can we get beyond our controversies? *Change, 24*(4) 9–11, 53.

3

Developing an Educational Partnership with a Neighborhood

Peggy S. Matteson

With careful planning, a neighborhood's residents, university faculty and students, and community providers may enter into a mutually beneficial educational experience. This chapter focuses on how faculty can begin to locate and develop clinical education opportunities for students in the community.

NEED FOR TRANSFORMATION

Traditionally, clinical assignments for nursing students have been developed within institutions that provide services to a number of patients in need of relatively short-term units of predictable care. Established curriculum dictates which nursing interventions are covered in which courses, and students are basically restricted to learning and then implementing the selected topic of care. To support this agenda, students are assigned to specific patients within an institution in a relatively focused manner so that the main disease or problem of the patient correlates with the concepts under study for that week or clinical rotation. The selection of course subjects and the approach to learning about them are determined by the faculty, with little or no consideration for the life experiences of students or patients. This system ensures students' conformity but doesn't meet the real needs of patients and their families.

As part of its participation in Boston's Center for Community Health, Education, Research, and Service (CCHERS), Northeastern University's College of Nursing has developed clinical learning experiences for its students based on facing the reality of life in the community and a problem-posing educational format. This concept of education strives for the emergence of consciousness and critical intervention based in the revealed reality of all participants (Freire, 1989). To successfully prepare to practice in the rapidly changing field of health care, students must not only become capable of lifetime learning but also be willing to derive their subject content from their own learning experiences. Moreover, the learning must be grounded in reality. Long-term involvement with a neighborhood of clients allows this to happen.

Developing a relationship with a neighborhood in order to simultaneously provide health services for residents while they participate in the experience of educating nursing students creates a shared partnership. The neighborhood residents and the health care providers already in place within the neighborhood agree to include students within the community of mutual care and concern. This is important for the students' learning process because to understand clients' behaviors the student must understand how the situation looked to them, what they thought they had to contend with, what alternatives they saw available to them. Students can understand the effects of opportunity structures, delinquent subcultures, social norms, and other commonly invoked explanations of behavior only by seeing them from the resident's point of view (Becker, 1966, pp. vi-vii).

To develop an educational partnership between the members of seemingly disparate settings, such as a college of nursing and a selected neighborhood, individuals of both locations need to work to develop a structure that enables all participants to interact and learn from each other. When the opportunity is provided for interaction, it becomes "the means by which men and women deal critically and creatively with reality and discover how to participate in the transformation of their world" (Freire, 1989, p. 15).

When the members of a university come into a neighborhood and learn about the problems from the residents, reality is continuously unveiled. This alternative focus fosters creativity, creates an interactive process in the development of the content of education, and enhances the students' development in the process of utilization of self. The representatives from the college of nursing (students and faculty) join with and learn from the residents as each brings her or his own expertise to the development of a mutual learning experience.

Field method is a generic term applied to the process of observing events in a natural situation. The development of a site for a field-method type of educational experience is, in many ways, similar to the location and establishment of a site for field research in any discipline. There are various steps that a faculty person goes through to successfully negotiate the establishment and maintenance of a neighborhood clinical site. First, potential neighborhoods must be identified and investigated. Then, relationships must be developed and access negotiated. Maintenance of access and the relationship between the affiliated parties is an ongoing process, as the needs and abilities to meet those needs are in constant flux within both the student population and neighborhood. Returning the same students to a particular neighborhood for longitudinal clinical experiences creates a sense of continuity for all participants and assists in this process.

Entry into this type of relationship is similar to the development of a relationship for field research. The optimal outcome is development of the student, teacher, provider, and consumer as collaborators with mutual goals and objectives and the potential for mutual benefits. Thus, clinical interventions are conceived and desired by all parties and collaboratively designed to provide information that would be used by both to effect a change in health status for individuals or groups within the neighborhood. Each party agrees to participate openly and reserves the option of withdrawing. Each has a vested interest in the success of this joint venture, and the motivation of each party is recognized and accepted by the other. Each is willing to openly acknowledge and discuss the grounds for continued participation in the relationship at any time (Reinharz, 1988).

IDENTIFYING A NEIGHBORHOOD

The word *neighborhood* is derived from Old English and means "near dweller." It evolved from the notion of extended family, and its residents are often seen as an extension of the family. Neighbors identify themselves as living near each other, and this provides a sense of acquaintance or even companionship. A sense of commonality leads them to differentiate themselves from those who live outside the area. The delineation of a neighborhood is based on the interaction of human beings who live near each other and distinguish themselves as coming from a certain area or having particular characteristics.

It is supportive of the students' educational experience to develop a partnership with members of an identifiable neighborhood because of a sense of collectiveness among the residents. Within this somewhat homogeneous milieu, students are exposed to generational and familial differences and learn how various facets of peoples' lives affect their own and others' health.

The idea of a neighborhood sometimes conjures images of a sharply circumscribed territory. However, whatever its substance, each neighborhood is continuous with other areas and bound up with them in various ways. Institutions within a neighborhood necessarily reach out toward other institutions and are penetrated or overlapped by them. There are generally no absolute spatial boundaries and no absolute beginnings or ends. Their parameters and properties are conceptual discoveries. However, even as one neighborhood blends into the next, there are some systematic ways to locate a neighborhood and determine just what the parameters might be.

Identifiable External Parameters of Neighborhoods

Specific neighborhoods, as defined by the residents, are created by virtue of a variety of natural or man-made factors. Faculty members must seek out a defined neighborhood, as it will be more unified and easier to work with in the development of educational programs. They must be alert to the fact that what may at first appear to be a neighborhood may be a population group that is divided by one or more of the following factors.

Physical Dividers

Groups of people may be isolated into neighborhoods by physical dividers, both natural and man made. Highways and rivers often prevent populations living within hundreds of yards of each other from interacting in a neighborly fashion. Within an urban environment an extensive business district or manufacturing district may create an artificial barrier between residential neighborhoods.

Access to public transportation and the lines the transportation then follows as it moves toward larger population centers not only facilitates but determines how people are able to interact with each other. Residents may find it easier to interact with others along the transportation lines than with those in closer proximity who live on a perpendicular to the lines.

Regulatory Dividers

The most obvious governmental parameters are state lines. Generally, it may be assumed that a neighborhood is located within a larger population unit within a single state. However, some neighborhoods have developed and maintained themselves while straddling a border, with residents situated in two different states.

Within states or regions governmental service agencies develop catchment areas that follow agency-specific divisional lines. For example, within a state the departments of public health and mental health may have designated different resource areas. This means that geographical neighbors may find themselves in the same catchment areas for some services and in different areas for other services.

Postal zip codes are another federal mechanism to delineate population groups, in this case to enhance postal delivery. Residents are readily able to identify themselves as living within a specific zip code area. In some places zip codes are used to label the socioeconomic level or cultural background of everyone living within a specific code.

Like zip codes, telephone numbers are used by people to identify the area in which they live. From an area code, which defines a large area, to the exchange number, which covers a small area, artificial lines are drawn and in some cases barriers are erected. When the boundary lines designating the service area for exchange numbers are drawn, sometimes population groups are divided, and residents may no longer telephone each other without incurring additional expense for the call. This financial factor then limits free communication and may cause a divide within a geographical neighborhood.

For data collection purposes the government has divided population areas into segments called census tracts; these were designed to collect and then apply statistical information to clearly defined areas. The use of census tracts has imposed artificial lines within population areas and has sometimes divided neighborhoods. For example, certain census tracts become labeled as needing specific services, whereas contiguous ones are not. Thus, governmental funding may become available for services within one tract but not for neighbors in an adjoining tract.

Voting districts are small residential areas that determine where a person votes. Residents within certain voting districts may be self-identified or identified in the media or by candidates for office as having certain characteristics, such as political affiliation, educational levels, economic status, or a particular view on how others should be treated, for example, a "liberal" or "conservative" view. When subgroups of a community view themselves as different from each other, they generally do not collaborate in the development of community goals or activities.

Cultural divergence, including language barriers and religious differences, also tend to separate groups of people within larger segments of the population. A sense of belonging and comfort often draws people of the same ethnic heritage together. Not only are they better able to communicate in their native tongue, but they are also more capable of supplying each other with goods and services supportive of their cultural heritage.

Internal Population Magnets

In areas close to people's homes, meeting places develop for business or pleasure. Recreational, religious, or governmental centers clustered together may create a focal point for neighborhood activity. Areas where these facilities cluster should be investigated as possible centers or hubs of an active neighborhood.

Recreational centers may cater to a single sex or a specific age group. They may be clubs with social agendas, athletic agendas, or a combination of both. The types and numbers of available facilities might reveal something about who is valued in the neighborhood, for example, more facilities for adult males than for women or adolescents.

Religious facilities may range from large edifices to storefront churches. Some buildings may be situated within the community but are not truly part of the community. For example, members of some churches or synagogues that were established many years ago may have moved out of the area and return only for worship services. Some facilities limit their community involvement to the hour(s) of weekly worship, whereas others make their facilities available for use by internal or external groups. This type of outreach provides a meeting place for the community regardless of attendees' religious affiliation.

Government buildings are generally located to serve the needs of residents. A cluster of one or two of these facilities, including public buildings such as post offices, schools, libraries. or public playgrounds, may form an active hub of a neighborhood.

Locating a Neighborhood for a Clinical Field Site

Area maps provide the first step in locating potential neighborhoods. By plotting the locations of external barriers and internal magnets to population groups within a selected region it is possible to identify various areas that might function as neighborhoods. Each neighborhood must then be evaluated in more detail and explored to determine (1) if the site is suitable for students; (2) if the size, population, cultural complexity, spatial scatter, health care resource, and the like provide sites with which to develop partnerships; and (3) if information is attainable about the place and the people so that an eventual plan may be developed to negotiate entry.

The importance of background interviewing and document research before faculty members actually move in to negotiate for specific neighborhood settings cannot be underestimated. The assessment process is similar to the participant observation format in qualitative research as the faculty member enters an unknown area to learn about its structure. "Participant observation . . . is nothing more than experiencing a setting, overcoming the difficulties of multidimensional, multipurpose interaction and recording one's observations" (Reinharz, 1988, p. 154).

The information that must be obtained in order to develop a successful plan of entry includes whom to approach and how, an understanding of the identities and power alignments of the elected and assumed leaders within the neighborhood, and the immediate interests and concerns of the leaders.

To gain a perspective about the present and possible future developments within the neighborhood, faculty members must learn its history and the activity focus of specific institutions within the area. This type of information may be skillfully garnered by browsing through a variety of sources, such as community newspapers, brochures, institutional histories, and public bulletin boards, as well as by informal conversations with neighborhood workers or residents.

Identifying the Neighborhood Leadership

Depending upon the size and structure of organizations within the neighborhood, the leaders may be elected, appointed, or assumed. There may be one primary community organizing group that encompasses the majority of community development activity, or there may be several, each involved with a specific segment of community welfare, such as a businessmen's association or a youth association. The leadership of each organization is selected by the mechanism defined in its bylaws.

Leadership within a community may also be assumed by a motivated individual. The individual may either earn the respect of others or cultivate a power base that allows her or him to be in control. In the process of assuming a leadership role and developing a power base, a leader may develop an organization to serve the needs of the individual and/or the community.

Because there may be differences in the motivation and activities of organizations as an outgrowth of their developmental histories, it helps to learn as much as possible about the chronology of development and the purpose of each identified community organization. It is also useful to determine how much crossover exists between members of the groups and how well the various organizations have worked together in the past.

Identifying leaders within a community is fairly easy. Their names appear in the community newspaper, in reports about an organization's activities, and also in announcements, such as posters and flyers, alerting the residents to activities and services provided by the group. Determining whether an individual is a respected leader or merely a figurehead is more difficult and requires a longer period of watching and listening at community gatherings.

ASSESSING A NEIGHBORHOOD AS A CLINICAL SITE

Once the parameters, demographics, and leadership scheme of a neighborhood are obtained, it becomes possible to make a preliminary determination of the area's potential as a clinical site. If the site looks feasible, further exploration is needed to determine what services are currently available, the origination of each service, who currently sponsors it, the actual providers of the service, the neighborhood's response to the specific service, and the current level of collaboration between services.

Services Currently Available

A walk through the neighborhood is one easy way to begin to ascertain what services are available. Facilities have identifying signs at their entrances and advertisements for others are posted on bulletin boards. To meet the needs of its residents, neighborhood services may be developed locally or imported into the community from other bases of operation. Local services tend to develop in a specific response to an actual community need; they are small in focus, funded through local fund-raising, run on a skimpy or nonexistent budget, and depend on a great deal of volunteer assistance. These services may range in scope from a single youth service program to a full service community health center.

Services imported from outside the neighborhood are broader in scope, developed to meet an expected need of a diverse population, and dependent on funding from the government, private grants, or appeals to people outside the community. These services may include elderly activities or day care, home visitation programs for new mothers or the otherwise homebound, affiliates of national organizations, outreach services both private and governmental, and educational and health care facilities.

Origination of Services

Exploring who identified the need for this resource and who brought this service to the residents are important steps in the assessment process. Services developed locally are usually designed to meet a need identified by community residents. Food pantries, used-clothing closets, neighborhood watch programs, and elderly phone visitation programs are examples. Each one is organized on the model of neighbor helping neighbor, usually to serve a specific, urgent, possibly short-term need. Local residents govern and control the organization. Because the base of control lies with the residents themselves, their leaders can decide if a partnership with nursing students would assist the neighborhood.

Services developed on a broader base and brought into the neighborhood may come in response to an observed or speculated need, a government funding allocation, or to an invitation from community leaders. The parameters of the organization's service agenda are determined by a governing body generally located outside the neighborhood, on a state, county, regional, or national level. Depending on the corporate structure, residents may or may not be represented in a meaningful manner on the governing board. Programs may therefore be externally generated and only open to local modification. This type of program may not have the flexibility or desire to integrate the clinical activities of nursing students.

Financial Support of Services

The basis of an organization's financial support often indicates the community's support of the group and the group's integration into and commitment to the community. Some organizations limit their funding base to the people whom they serve and rely strongly on in-kind or volunteer support. Others expand their basis of support to include donations from individuals and groups outside the organization or even outside the neighborhood.

Financial support from outside the neighborhood may come from public or private sources or a combination of both. As an organization, such as a youth group or a neighborhood health center, grows, it usually begins to incorporate external fund-raising as a major piece of its activity in order to meet the clients' requests.

Some organizations are initially funded by an external source, either public or private, to develop a program to meet a specific community need. Once the project is started, the funding usually stops, and the project must become self-sustaining. Organizations developed in this manner may or may not be able to continue once the initial funding ceases.

Based on these considerations it is important to determine the type and duration of the funding commitment of an organization. Organizations with funding difficulties are less comfortable with incorporating students into their programs if they feel that the students will require extra time and effort from their staffs. If, however, leaders feel that the students will bring additional assistance to the provided services, they may value them as much as volunteers. Access to an organization and its clients is therefore enhanced when a long-term commitment is made by the college of nursing to become part of the service network of a neighborhood or of a specific organization. The students and faculty are more likely to be viewed as collaborators in the efforts rather than additional users of resources.

Providers of Services

Providers of services or care within health care agencies differ a great deal from one neighborhood to the next. To varying degrees agencies attempt to include members of the neighborhood at some level. This policy contributes credibility to the agency and makes it more approachable, integrating the organization into the neighborhood and serving as a role model, while providing a realistic grounding in the actual needs of the residents.

When members of the community do not have the interest or the expertise to fill certain positions within the health care agency, the next supportive strategy is to employ members of the same cultural group who live outside the neighborhood. They usually bring an understanding of the culture to their interactions and provide a degree of role modeling for their clients. Nevertheless, just because an individual is of the same cultural background as the client, an automatic understanding between them cannot be assumed. Individuals raised in different neighborhoods, at different times, and with possibly different expectations may be very dissimilar. However, with sensitivity and caring, bridges can be built and relationships developed when the commonality of ancestral heritage provides a solid base.

A third alternative found in the staffing of an agency is the employment of outsiders who may be different culturally, economically, and/or educationally from the clients they serve. Although this type of staffing may be necessary because of needed expertise, it does not facilitate relationship building between the agency and the residents of the neighborhood.

To be successful in meeting the needs of the neighborhood and the expertise needs of the agency, it is often necessary to develop a staff with a mix of providers. For these same reasons, agencies are also more receptive to incorporating a mix of nursing students within their operations. Nursing students can provide role models not only to the young residents of the neighborhood but also to other employees of the agency.

Neighborhood's Response

A neighborhood's response to an agency depends on how people view the services provided, how they view the providers, and how they picture themselves in relation to the agency. If the residents feel that the agency has developed from within their midst and they have a sense of ownership, they will be much more involved in its utilization than if they view it as imposed from the outside. A neighborhood's interaction with an agency can be determined by the extent of the use of its services, the participation by residents on its boards and communities, and the comments of residents in informal conversation.

Answers to the following questions help determine a resident's regard for an agency: Are they aware the agency exists? Are they familiar with the services it provides? Do they know anyone who works there? Have they ever sought assistance from the agency? Do they know of anyone who has? What were their experiences? Responses to these questions will also help determine the possible degree to which nursing students will learn about and interact with residents if they become affiliated with the agency.

Interaction between Services

In deciding which agencies to approach, the faculty must also consider the amount of interaction between agencies. Some work collaboratively with other providers, each filling a niche, and yet all working toward a common purpose.

Other agencies set boundaries and maintain minimal interaction or collaboration with other organizations. A primary affiliation with such a group will limit the development of future associations for students within a community and severely limit their learning about the many facets of a neighborhood.

NEGOTIATING ENTRY

After the necessary information is collected and analyzed, the next step is an informal inquiry into selected health care institutions within the neighborhood. Selection criteria include the following: the agency is successful and has a positive impact, it cooperates with other agencies, and it is respected and utilized by the residents. Agency use by residents implies a client-focused rather than provider-focused agenda.

The first visit by faculty members may be structured to send up a trial balloon about their desire to incorporate students into the health care activities of this neighborhood. This visitation process will include both the gathering of additional data about the site and a test of receptivity. A genuine appreciative interest in the neighborhood and its residents on the part of faculty is critical. Even the most impressive credentials will open only certain doors (and could possibly close others).

The quality of the response is determined by residents' and providers' prior interactions with researchers or educators who have come in with their own agendas, intruded into subjects' privacy, disrupted their perceptions, utilized false pretenses, manipulated the relationship, and given little or nothing in return (Reinharz, 1988). Genuine rapport, which will create the most conducive educational environment, is established when the community and agency leaders, and then the residents accept the faculty and students for their personal qualities rather than formal status).

Techniques used to make a formal contact, for the approach

and engagement of a working relationship depend on the preference of the educator. Some use the phone easily; some prefer writing first and then following up with a visit. In planning the initial contact faculty members must keep the hierarchy of the institution in mind. If they enter with the permission of the "chief" at the site of care, they are in a better position to continue to negotiate further entry into all aspects of the organization. If initial access is granted by an off-site administrator, entry into the actual programs of the facility and interactions with clients are still controlled by the person in charge of the site.

The following strategies will help faculty members gain entry into neighborhood organizations:

- Bargain for a role for yourself and your students within the realm of the organization.
- Learn from the organization's leaders what their needs and desires are concerning the health of the community.
- Explain to the leadership how you and your students might be able to meet one or several of those needs.
- Start small and gradually expand later if you desire.
- Set mutually developed objectives with the leadership for both community participants and nursing students.

If faculty members fulfill their initial commitments, site expansion will come more easily.

The development of a neighborhood clinical site at a senior day program provides an example of this process. A day facility for senior citizens is located in a storefront, one of many established and run by municipal services. Seniors walk to or are bused to the location. There is an on-site director who develops and coordinates the activities within the overall framework determined by the organization's administration.

Gaining entry to this site was initiated by the faculty member's walking into the facility and meeting the on-site director. An explanation of the desire to bring nursing students into the neighborhood and the collaborative nature of the relationship caught the interest of the director. She provided a description of the activities of the program and started to think of ways in which the students could help the clients. Her one concern was whether

her boss, the program administrator, would approve of this collaborative effort.

Based on the needs of her clients and the developing abilities of the students, an activity plan was negotiated that specified the roles of the senior citizens and the nursing students. This provided clarity to each of the leaders within this new working relationship, as well as a written plan for the off-site administrator. With a plan formulated, the director approached the program's administrator for permission. Approval was gained, and the director was praised by the administration for her foresight and initiative in developing a new service for her clients.

The initial commitment of student time to this facility was limited to a specific activity: individual health histories of the clients. Successful achievement led to an easing of restrictions and additional access. Activities were no longer subject to the approval of the administrator. With continued interaction, greater understanding developed between the director and the faculty member of the college of nursing. With input from the clients and students, other successful activities have been planned. By starting small, fulfilling the commitment, and then gradually expanding the number and type of interactions, the possibility of a continuing relationship slowly became a reality.

Meet with Providers

Because the students will be collaborating with the actual providers of services and viewing them as role models, it is important for faculty member to learn how providers view students, as well as the clients and their needs. Through conversations it is possible to ascertain the views and beliefs of providers. Do they enjoy their work and convey a sense of accomplishment? Do they have a knowledge base of the cultural needs of their clients? Are they understanding of the obstacles that residents encounter when seeking care? Attitudinal factors, as well as skill development, are important lessons that students learn through interactions with providers, and the faculty must ensure that the lessons are appropriate.

Providers need a brief outline concerning the students' communication, critical thinking, and therapeutic abilities as they start and then progress through each course. Those outside academe often forget that students have specific objectives that must be met within each course and that their professional development is relatively sequential and goal-oriented. The faculty member must explain the focus of the clinical experience for each course.

After supplying this information the faculty member can discuss ways to incorporate the abilities of the students. Concrete examples agreed on by providers and faculty members are most beneficial as they mutually negotiate the role of the student. Because faculty members enter through the auspices of the head of the organization, they have underlying bargaining rights. Nevertheless, how well the students are received depends on whether the providers come to view them as another chore forced upon them or as collaborators in care.

During the collaborative development of students' roles, the provider serves as the expert on the needs of the clients, as well as the facility, and the university faculty member is the expert on the learning needs of the students. The challenge is for the students to take on activities that meet the needs of residents and the facility and simultaneously meet their own needs.

Ongoing Concerns

Gaining entry is a continuous process of establishing and developing relationships, not only with the director of the program or agency but also with a variety of other personnel. Successful negotiation through the front door does not necessarily guarantee full cooperation with students from all within the organization. Maintaining a viable partnership within a relatively complex human organization is a continuous process and requires the efforts of all involved. Individual interactions are necessary to develop true support for the educational efforts of each person within the organization. The interaction may be as simple as the faculty member or student sharing a mutual interest with another employee, or it may take the form of an in-depth negotiated session with a leader of a subdivision within the agency. Even when relationships with individuals in particular roles are well established, they must be renegotiated because of the relatively frequent changes within the organization's staff.

Providers respond differently to students. Some may feel overwhelmed that they must deal with students in addition to their other duties. Some may not feel comfortable as role models to students. On the other hand, some may feel neglected if they do not have the opportunity to interact with students.

Because the students' needs may not be met exclusively within one agency, several entries may be necessary, each at a different site within the neighborhood. Faculty members must move slowly in the sequencing of this activity, as the agencies may not be supportive of this. Setting priorities for partnerships helps to keep options open. As faculty members approach and gain entry to a site, they can ask for suggestions from their new associates about which sites to approach next. This prevents them from placing themselves between two competing sites, with the risk of losing both, and allows the first site to facilitate entry into additional sites. In a mutually voluntary and negotiated entry, the host agency holds the options to continue or end the relationship at any time, so the development of clinical sites with a constant awareness of intraagency and interagency politics is always necessary.

WORKING WITH COMMUNITY ORGANIZATIONS

To develop a clinical site with a neighborhood, it is easier, but not required, that a community health center be present. A variety of additional or alternative clinical sites may be found in any neighborhood. Each has the potential to meet learning objectives of students at various levels of ability, and by combining sites students can meet a wide variety of learning needs. Each potential clinical site maintains an organizational head as well as providers. At some sites these roles may be filled by the same person. The experts from whom the students may learn are administrators, providers, and users of the organization's services. To successfully negotiate entry for students, faculty members must be able to present ideas about the potential roles students might fill.

Identification of potential sites is limited only by the imagination. Examples of some apparent as well as less common sites are provided to facilitate the exploration process.

Day Care Centers

Whether a day care center serves children from infancy through preschool or just segments of that population, it provides an opportunity for students to observe the stages of growth and development, assess the health behaviors of children, provide health screening, and learn the process of interacting with and teaching children of various ages, their families, and staff members. Entrance is gained through the director of the program, and development of students' learning experiences usually occurs with a teacher of a particular class. The teachers are the experts in the area of childhood education and the process of interacting with children. They are specifically expert on the individuality of each of their charges and on cultural diversity. Staff members help nursing students understand the normal variations and how to approach and teach children.

The knowledge and skills that the nursing students bring focus on health assessment, including screening, health education, and first aid. If chronically ill children are part of the population, nursing students are able to offer specialized, in-depth education for staff. Few day care centers offer the services of a school nurse to their clientele, so students can take on many elements of that role for one class or the whole center.

Schools

Neighborhood schools may include elementary, middle, and/or high schools. Even though the schools may all be part of the same system, each is a world unto itself, and entrance is gained only by permission of the principal. In some cases the principal may also require permission from the superintendent of schools or the school committee.

The health care interventions provided by the nursing students depend on the programs provided within the school, the age level, and the population served. Some schools maintain classrooms for special-needs students, allowing nursing students to develop interactions with a variety of handicapped children. Other providers within the facility may include a school nurse, a speech therapist, and an occupational or physical therapist. Each provider may share her or his expertise with nursing students and allow them to develop interventions with their young clients.

Regardless of the programs already offered within the schools, nursing students may assess individual or group needs, develop a plan to meet those needs, and then provide appropriate interventions. Just as within the day care center, the classroom teacher is the expert on her or his particular age group in general and the charges within that room in particular. The nursing students offer their developing health care expertise to work within a collaborative process. The nursing students learn how to interact effectively with students from various cultural backgrounds and present topics so that effective learning occurs. With assistance, students can initiate health screening, immunization clinics, and violence prevention programs.

Schoolteachers generally maintain a high level of concern for the health and well-being of their students. Yet because of limited funding and personnel, many potential projects are never undertaken. When nursing students wish to care for the health needs of the students in exchange for learning from classroom experts, teachers are usually more than happy to welcome them.

Senior Citizen Programs

A variety of programs exist for senior citizens. Some are run as social clubs for those elderly who are interested in interacting with others and are able to leave their homes. Others are established around nutritional programs, in which the elderly are brought together for a meal at noontime and some degree of socialization or activity. A third type of program serves those who need daily care yet are competent enough to not require admission to a nursing home.

Each type of program has a director, on- or off-site. Introductory advances should be made to the person in charge at the specific neighborhood site of interest to explore the purpose of the program, the number and type of clientele, the services currently provided, and the potential benefit to the clients from interacting with the nursing students. If different employees or volunteers are responsible for various aspects of the program, faculty members will have to engage each one of them individually after receiving approval and introduction from the director. Programs tend to be planned with no free time available to the clients within the day's structure. To arrange for students to collaborate with providers or participate in various segments of the program, faculty members must make sure the leader of that segment understands the purpose and value of the students' interactions.

Students gain a number of insights during interactions with the elderly. Many students have grown up away from extended family and are not aware that most of the aged live independently within the community. Using open-ended questions, students may conduct a cultural assessment, a nutritional assessment, or a health history. Listening to the elderly describe their health histories, students learn much about how adults care for themselves so that they may reach old age. By participating with the clients in various activities, such as modified aerobics or craft activities, they are able to assess range of motion and motor skills.

Depending on the focus of the program and the assessed needs of the clients, such interventions as health teaching, nutritional status evaluation, medication checks, flu clinics, home visits, hypertension and cholesterol screening, and domestic violence prevention, as well as care requiring more technical skills, are all possible. The longer the students are associated with a specific group of elderly people, the more complex their involvement in care may become.

Courts

The judicial system provides an interesting opportunity for students to observe and assess members of a community under extreme stress. Some judges, especially in family court, keep a nurse on staff to assess the health and mental status of those scheduled to appear before them. The nurse is also responsible for home visits and for evaluating the potential outcomes of the possible decisions that a judge may make. Collaborating with a nurse working in this capacity provides advanced students with the opportunity to use a number of critical thinking, communication, and therapeutic intervention skills.

When a nurse is not available in this capacity, students are still capable of learning from court interactions. Students may be matched with the clerks who staff the front lines and respond to residents' stress reduction or knowledge needs as they file restraining orders. Other experts who may share time and knowledge with students are the client advocates or support persons who accompany women through court procedures after a rape or domestic assault.

Access to the court system can occur through a judge who employs a nurse or through the clerks servicing claimants. Only through observing the system and focusing on the development of contacts can faculty members assess the potential of the local court as a clinical site.

Occupational Health

The residents of a neighborhood are often employed within the same geographical location. In keeping with *Nursing's Agenda for Healthcare Reform* (American Nurses Association, 1991), to take health care services to where the people are, students may become involved in providing health care services within places of employment.

Generally, very large firms maintain a clinic for employees, and the company's employee health nurse can be a suitable collaborator for students. In smaller businesses, students working more independently may become involved in assessing the health and safety needs of employees and then developing programs to meet these needs.

Access to this population is through the local head of the company. If faculty members begin by providing a short summary of the health care services students may offer, company leaders will be able to conceptualize the value of student's services to the health of the employees.

Library

The community library, usually not considered a site for health care, can provide several creative possibilities. Bulletin boards are placed in prominent places for the public to view. They offer information about activities within the community and can be used by students who wish to display health care information and announcements of programs. As a public meeting place, the library often provides programs for various constituencies and may welcome health care programs presented by students as an extension of its community service.

Access to bulletin boards or meeting space is gained through the director of the library. Library employees can offer information about patterns of use, the informational interests and needs of their clients, and the programs they feel will be best received by the members of the neighborhood.

The library itself is the repository of possible information clients might seek out to gain a better understanding about health matters and disease processes. Students can gain a better understanding of the abilities of clients to do this type of research if they themselves attempt to use the facilities.

Visiting Nurse Associates

Visiting nurse programs have been in existence for a number of years. Originally an outgrowth of neighborhood nursing, they now are usually organized around a community larger than a single neighborhood. Services are paid for by government programs, such as Medicare and Medicaid, and other types of health insurance. Nurses tend to care for patients in their homes within a fairly broad area. Students learn about many aspects of nursing practice when they collaborate with a nurse during home visits.

Accessing a visiting nurse service as a clinical experience for nursing students in a selected neighborhood is not always easy. Residents often know of nurses coming into the neighborhood, and a faculty member can approach the visiting nurse and explain the students' role within the neighborhood. If the nurse is receptive, a meeting with the director is the next step. Many nurses are hesitant to take on a nursing student because they fear students will slow them down in their visits and interfere with the patient-nurse relationship. If faculty members can address these two issues immediately by explaining how the nursing students will be of assistance, they may be fortunate enough to obtain a trial placement. Then, as the value of a nursing student becomes more apparent, placements will grow.

Religious Organizations

Churches, synagogues, and other facilities for organized religious services provide various possibilities for students within a neighborhood. Publicizing health promotion activities within a neighborhood is one possibility. For example, announcements made by the clergy from the pulpit or in the organization's publications will reach a great many of the residents within the neighborhood.

The facilities of the organization are also potential sites for a variety of health care interventions. Because religious centers are situated within a populated area and are considered safe havens, residents are more apt to attend a health screening program, an immunization clinic, a nutritional program, a series of educational sessions, or any other needed intervention there. The range and scope of the program are limited only by the needs of the residents and the abilities of the students.

Individual client identification is also possible through the pastor of the congregation. Leaders are often aware of parishioners of all ages who would benefit from simple to complex nursing interventions within their homes. The recipients of care can be identified and initial contact made through the organization's office. To develop this type of program, faculty members must gain the trust of the clergy and make them aware of the health screening (i.e., blood pressure) and health promotion services (i.e. blood sugar testing, skin care, immunizations) that nursing students are capable of providing and the available backup resources. Appropriate confidentiality must be assured. The parishioner must also trust the students and value the health care interventions to be offered. With this type of program the student becomes closely involved with one neighborhood family, allowing family members to assist in the student's acculturation. As students develop though the nursing program, they are able to offer more complex health care services to clients.

Understanding the benefit of an alliance with nurses, some churches have a parish nurse program in place. Models vary from one congregation to the next. Nurses may work full-time, part-time, or a few hours a week. They may be paid by hospitals or churches or work as volunteers. Some are in partnership with schools of nursing. They focus on health education, personal health counseling, coordinating volunteers, referrals to community resources, and the integration of faith and health. When nurses are certified in advanced practice, they often provide more direct care in church-based clinics, private homes, nursing homes, or even hospitals. The great advantage of parish nurses is that they know and are known by the population they serve (Chandler, 1994). Students can provide a variety of services to parishioners while developing a holistic perspective of care.

Community Outreach Programs

Within the services provided to members of a neighborhood are a variety of outreach programs staffed by nurses and other health care workers, health educators, youth workers, recreation leaders, and/or community advocates. Depending upon the specific purpose and implementation of a program, it may provide assessment and intervention experiences that can serve a variety of educational objectives and professional developmental levels.

Funding availability usually determines the initiatives being developed and the programs currently functioning. Federal and state concerns generally focus on the elderly; teenage pregnancy; violence, both domestic and street; substance abuse; and acquired immune deficiency syndrome (AIDS).

Elderly

Homebound individuals, whether elderly or invalid, receive visitation services for assessment and socialization or to meet basic needs. For example, a program such as Meals-on-Wheels provides a hot meal distributed by volunteers. On a regular basis the organizing agency arranges home visits to assess the client's status, inquire about the acceptability of the food (which may be a problem for culturally diverse populations), and determine if other services are needed. Students, working with an agency representative, can assist with many of these functions while learning the needs and frustrations of those unable to easily leave the confines of their home.

Another outreach service helps the older or elderly adult who is faced with the task of raising one or more grandchildren. This is not a person who agrees to provide child care for a part of each day but one who has accepted the full legal and sometimes financial responsibility for child rearing. The situation develops when an adult son or daughter is no longer capable of caring for his or her children as a result of continuing substance abuse, incarceration, or some other serious problem or when the parent has died.

In some instances a grandparent has turned to the court to seek custody of a grandchild(ren) removed from a parent. To provide the grandchildren with a continuation of familial care the grandparent(s) takes on the task. Limited in financial and energy resources, grandparents may be served by a program such as Raising Our Children's Children (ROCC), started in Dorchester, Massachusetts by Harriet Jackson-Lyons, a grandmother in such a situation. ROCC provides its members, aged 32 to over 80, with supportive care, simultaneously addressing grief resolution, parenting, and aging issues. Whether they are comfortable with developing and providing parenting interventions or caring for the elderly, students learn from grandparents how to best combine these areas into a holistic approach to care.

Teenage Pregnancy

Pregnancy among teenagers is both unintended and intended. Community-based initiatives to decrease the number of pregnancies have been developed and incorporated into programs at youth clubs, after-school programs, and organized gatherings of adolescents sponsored by community groups. Once the nursing students have gained the trust of the teens and developed a relationship with them, they will learn the factors that motivate abstinence and sexual activity and their concerns about each. In ways that fit into the reality of the teen's world, students can find many opportunities to provide teaching, screening, and appropriate referrals that can influence behaviors.

Most teenage women who choose to raise a child need a variety of supportive services, over and above social services. In response to that need a community outreach program may involve a group such as Supportive Sisters, developed in Boston. Women who have themselves experienced adolescent parenting are paired for one-to-one contact with parenting adolescents. In the Supportive Sisters program an older woman provides emotional support, positive reinforcement, practical information, modeling of parenting skills, and periodic companionship within a judgment-free environment. Nursing students have found it beneficial to organize and develop supportive services for the older women, planning educational sessions for them as they too progress in their parenting roles, and organizing monthly or bi-weekly forums for group discussions or educational programs.

Violence Prevention

Violence, both on the streets and in the home, is a concern of most neighborhoods. The community members' response to these issues varies. Some programs are directed at decreasing gang violence through the development of alternative activities; some communities have developed educational programs, hotlines, and in some cases, a safe house for abused women. Often reluctant to bring "outsiders" into these programs, community members may initially block the involvement of students. As the students' presence in the neighborhood becomes increasingly acceptable and their abilities come to be valued, involvement in this area of nursing care may become a possibility.

AIDS Programs

Programs for persons who test positive for the human immuno-deficiency virus (HIV) or have developed AIDS are available in many communities. Some programs also include a focus on other sexually transmitted diseases. Students may become involved with transmission-prevention programs or with identification, counseling, and care of those dealing with the disease. The prevention of transmission is based on education. To be effective, the educational intervention must be culturally acceptable in both format and language. Students may collaborate with funded personnel, many of whom are health educators but not nurses, and representatives from various cultures within the neighborhood to develop a sensitive and effective educational program. In attracting and facilitating neighborhood residents to participate in planning, implementing the project, ensuring that the health care information is complete and accurate, and evaluating the program to justify continued funding, students develop a variety of skills.

Community outreach programs designed to offer services to those with AIDS also provide learning opportunities for students. Working within testing sites, undergoing training as counselors, providing one-to-one services within buddy programs, and developing and presenting holistic health education programs for persons with AIDS (PWAs), are possible options that can be investigated.

The level of student involvement within such specialties should be based on students' areas of interest and the level of their developing professional abilities. Many opportunities provided by community outreach programs require a longitudinal time commitment so that students can develop a level of specialized knowledge and become able to provide more complex care.

SUMMARY

Changes in the health care system mandate that nursing students be prepared with clinical experiences that ready them for future roles. When a faculty member is challenged to develop clinical sites outside the hospital and traditional ambulatory settings, there are methods to facilitate the process and its success. An unusual but very effective mechanism is to develop a collaborative educational relationship between a limited number of students from each educational level and the members of a neighborhood. With each member of the coalition, whether university faculty members, nursing student, provider, or resident, considered an expert in his or her field learning becomes a mutually beneficial experience based in reality.

The process of identification and investigation of a possible neighborhood with which to create such an alliance is much like developing a site for field research. Becoming aware of the factors that facilitate the development and maintenance of a neighborhood as a learning environment is a necessary beginning to locating a viable site.

The interest of the neighborhood's leaders and service providers must be obtained in order to gain entry. The focus and scope of practice of various health care providers offer a place to initially develop students' learning experiences. A collaborating neighborhood provides a variety of educational experiences, opportunities for students to develop longitudinal relationships with clients and learn from a variety of experts, the development of individualized interests and professional skills, and professional service to those in need of health care.

REFERENCES

American Nurses Association. (1991). *Nursing's agenda for healthcare reform*. Kansas City: Author.

Becker, H. (1966). Introduction. In C. Shaw (Ed.), *The Jack Roller: A delinquent boy's own story*. Chicago: University of Chicago Press. (Originally published 1929)

Chandler, E. (1994, June). Parish nursing. *BayState Nurse News*, p. 5.

Freire, P. (1989). *Pedagogy of the oppressed*. New York: Continuum.

Reinharz, S. (1988). *On Becoming a social scientist*. New Brunswick, NJ: Transaction.

4

Introducing Students to the Neighborhood

Barbara R. Kelley

If nurses are to be prepared to care for people in the present and future changing health care system, they must understand the dynamics of and be comfortable working in the everyday world of the patient, the place the patient came from, and the place he or she will return to. Students prepared in this way will realize that knowledge of the environment is essential information in planning for and providing health care to an individual or a family. This information allows the student to recognize and utilize the neighborhood supports essential for individual and family well-being. And equally as important, it enables the students to become privy to the physical and emotional destabilization that occurs in families and individuals when the neighborhood is no longer able to fulfill its fundamental function for society.

LEARNING ABOUT A NEIGHBORHOOD

How do students learn about a neighborhood? There are many ways to gather data about a neighborhood and its inhabitants. The process is a dynamic and interactive one that involves the collection, sifting, and cataloging of information. Chapter 3 touched on many aspects of a neighborhood that faculty members must be concerned about when selecting educational sites and experiences for students. This chapter will highlight and explore some of the aspects that students need to focus on when they are engaged in learning about and working within a neighborhood.

Perhaps the best way to learn about a neighborhood is total immersion. Living, shopping, making friends and acquaintances, playing, and doing business in a neighborhood offer a broad range of subjective and objective learning experiences. But this level of involvement may not be possible or even necessary for nursing students to understand the role of the neighborhood in health care and how it fits into the larger system of human interaction. Faculty members at Northeastern University College of Nursing have found some useful tools that provide students with the opportunity to (1) learn about the neighborhood's history, (2) become involved with neighborhood groups, (3) listen to the people in the neighborhood, and (4) participate in health care with the neighborhood health care providers.

HISTORY OF THE NEIGHBORHOOD

Taking the history of a neighborhood can be likened to taking the history of an individual. The neighborhood is presented by a resident to the students in much the same way as a patient is. Through a walking or bus tour of the area, students begin to familiarize themselves with the demographics. The tour offers an opportunity for each student to form an impression of the neighborhood. It is an opportunity to collect both subjective and objective information (Appendix E). As students actually see the physical layout, they hear the sounds, languages, and idioms of the area. They smell the smells, taste the tastes, and get a feel for the people, places, and things that combine to make up the neighborhood.

Because neighborhoods mean different things to different people, it is useful for students to share their observations and feelings with each other and with representatives from the neighborhood. By doing this, students will understand that there is not just one true view of a neighborhood, that individuals see different things and view them differently, that there are, in fact, multiple realities.

During the tour, historical facts are discussed and historical sites observed. How was this particular neighborhood born? What were the antecedents? Has this particular neighborhood always been part of the larger city or community from its inception? Was it carved out of another area and annexed later, or does it stand alone without ties or allegiances to a larger whole? Was it made up of groups of people who found themselves in close geographic proximity, or did it have its beginnings as a "gateway neighborhood" to newly arriving immigrants? Did it grow up around employment opportunities, fishing, shoe factories, mills? This historical perspective provides an insight into the traditions and underlying values that originally brought people together.

The intervening history provides insights into the status quo. Were there any major surgeries in the past, that is, was any part of the neighborhood divided by a major highway or other construction; was its sense of cohesion and identity interrupted? Had any accidents or disasters, natural or man-made, such as floods or fires, ever changed the face of the neighborhood? Tracing the subsequent growth and development of the neighborhood and becoming familiar with the changes driven by social, economic, political, cultural, and religious circumstances give students a sense of the glue that holds the neighborhood together. It gives them a feeling for the neighborhood's strength and resilience. And it exposes weak spots that may require reinforcement or realignment.

Based on their introductory experiences, students begin to realize that a neighborhood is a dynamic entity. They come to understand that changes within a neighborhood, whether positive or negative, define not only the neighborhood but also the individuals within.

COMPONENTS OF A NEIGHBORHOOD

This initial overview is the first of many. Students are expected to record these impressions and observations for later reflection. As they become more familiar with the neighborhood and its people, they can review their first impressions and gain an understanding of how their own preconceptions may have influenced what they saw and what they missed. They begin to appreciate the powerful and often misleading nature of first impressions.

Although the definition of a neighborhood may be elusive, it is important for the student to understand that a neighborhood is a place and it is people. By using their senses, students begin to perceive how the inhabitants experience themselves and their surrounding environment. Is there a strong sense of cohesion, of openness, or is the neighborhood somewhat scattered or closed and withdrawn? What are the homes like? Are they large apartment buildings, two- or three-family dwellings, or single homes? Are they in good repair, painted, with fences and grass or flowers? Is there trash around or graffiti in evidence? Do the owners of the buildings live in the neighborhood, or are they absentee landlords? What is the ratio of public to private housing?

The Human Climate

One thing for students to consider is the Sociability Quotient (Warren & Warren, 1977). This is a measure of "neighborliness," the willingness of neighbors to exchange greetings or visits. It is a reflection of the openness of the individuals to accept and share space with others. The students need to look around and pay attention to who is out and moving around the neighborhood. Do people stop to greet one another, share a conversation? Is there evidence of young families with carriages or strollers? Are there children playing or teenagers in groups on corners? How many schools are there, and where are they located? Are there playgrounds, and how do they look, well kept or full of debris? Are there youth centers and places to play sports?

Are elderly people in evidence and are they alone or with others? Can they walk safely? What kind of places are there for people to congregate? Are there social clubs for men, and if so, how many? If the number of social clubs for men outnumber the clubs for young people, this implies something about the neighborhood, its identity, and values.

In the overall assessment of the area, students are helped to understand that the neighborhood is made up of individuals who are or were part of a family. One question to consider is the concept of family in the neighborhood. Are the people more comfortable with the traditional model of family, or are they open and accepting of alternative family patterns? Are single parents supported with day care and after-school programs? What would happen to a gay or lesbian family? How many household heads are grandparents?

Cultural assessment is also critical. What impact have changing demographics had on the neighborhood? How have the neighborhood and its people adjusted to these changes? How are cultural beliefs and practices expressed in the neighborhood? Does everyone share the same dominant culture, or is there evidence of cultural diversity? Are there stores that cater to specific cultural needs? Do signs display languages other than English? Where are they located? Is there a small cultural enclave within a neighborhood? How would students learn about strengths and problems? It is important to consider what a neighborhood means to newly arriving immigrant groups. People from developing countries often come from small, homogeneous villages. Although they may live within an identified American community, their ideas of neighbor and neighborhood may traverse the traditional geographic boundaries. They may feel more comfortable seeking services, help, and support elsewhere.

The Political Climate

To understand how thing happen, how things "get done," students need to appreciate neighborhood politics. Is the neighborhood a small, autonomous community unto itself or does the overall governance come from a city hall that is far removed in space and time? Affiliation with a larger unit may be a source of pride or a point of contention. Whatever the case, it is important to define the links to those in power. Does the connection flow both ways, or is it only from outside officials in? If the larger governing unit is in charge of essential services, how do the neighborhood people make their voices heard? Who are local leaders with political connections; how strong are they; and can the neighbors depend on them for help and guidance? Is the process of choosing local representatives open and representative of the various groups, or are there old-time political families that hand power down from generation to generation?

Interest groups serve many purposes in the political process. One of these is to collectively empower people who are often unheard and unnoticed. Students begin to learn who these groups are, the reasons for their existence, and how successful they are in putting forth their agenda. Grass-roots movements have been successful in securing and implementing legal rights for African-Americans, workers, and women, to name a few. It is essential for nursing students, who are future health care professionals, to understand that community organizing has the power to transform society (Rubin & Rubin, 1992). The very work of organizing helps individuals develop skills, a sense of efficacy and competence, and a sense of self-worth. Neighborhood health centers, in partnership with the neighborhoods, can address problems such as lack of affordable housing, drug abuse, discrimination, violence, and lack of access to health care. This kind of community organizing creates a capacity for democracy and sustained social change.

Neighborhoods are also strengthened by the investment of private concerns and organizations. Learning that there is little to no public-private interface is as important as finding out what does exist. Power accrues to people and groups that are successful. The existence of private input such as time, money, and space, enhances neighborhood esteem and encourages further development.

The Socioeconomic Climate

A neighborhood tour gives the student a sense of the socioeconomic climate of the area. Is this an upper-class or middle-class neighborhood with single-family dwellings? Are the streets in good repair and free of litter? Is this an old neighborhood with multiple family dwellings? Are the buildings all alike, or do some display individual characteristics, evidence of traditions that have been handed down? Are churches and temples apparent and welcoming, and are they representative of the area's population? Students are told to look for any indications that the neighborhood shares a sense of pride in its accomplishments and the contributions of its inhabitants. Are there any banners proclaiming "community pride day" or "clean up our neighborhood day?" Do the storefronts display posters or invitations to neighborhood dances, concerts, or benefits for causes? Are neighborhood children's or youth groups' contributions celebrated in poster or picture displays?

It is also important to recognize any homeless or transient population on the streets. Students should look for any services in the way of shelters or soup kitchens that the neighborhood offers. What is the general feeling or attitude displayed toward "street people"? Are they ignored, or are they victimized by individuals or groups in the neighborhood? Is there a sense that any of the homeless people are from the neighborhood, so "we must take care of our own"?

The economic viability of a neighborhood is an important part of the assessment. Is this neighborhood a "bedroom community" for some larger urban city or suburban industrial enclave, or is it a small cosmos unto itself? Students are directed to pay attention to the businesses. Are they small, owner-run stores? Is there a sense that they are busy, that they cater to the needs of the neighborhood and its diversity? Are there large food stores within walking distance or only small, expensive convenience stores? Are there pharmacies near by, and what are the operating hours? It is also important to find out if local industries or businesses provide the area people with employment. Students must also have a sense of conflicting and competing demands faced by the neighborhood and its inhabitants. Do the businesses and industries that form a solid economic base interfere with and harm the neighborhood environmentally? Are they a source of pollution, and how is that conflict framed and addressed? Equally important to know, is this economic base a viable and sustainable one. If businesses or industries are closing or moving away, what are the potential problems for the neighborhood?

The obvious signs of neighborhood pride, both individual and collective, help students understand the concept of empowerment. Who is in control of the neighborhood? How powerful are people who share the same values, and how willing are they to work together? And what happens when the neighborhood loses control of itself, becomes dysfunctional?

Legal and Illegal Activity

Does the neighborhood appear safe? Are there a good mix of people out and about? Do people walk quickly with their heads down, or do they stroll about, exchanging looks and greetings? Are there small groups of people in doorways or on street corners? Does it look as if there is any drug activity? Do the adults seem concerned with childrens' behavior, admonishing them to be careful or observing them at play?

An important part of any assessment is the observer's subjective feelings. Students can ask themselves how they feel in the neighborhood; are they comfortable walking around, or do they feel hesitant and wary? Are police visible walking the beat or directing traffic, or are they at the police station or in patrol cars? Is the neighborhood full of traffic or relatively quiet? Are drivers courteous; do they stop for pedestrians or speed through the streets? Where are the fire stations and how up-to-date is the equipment? Are fire hydrants well cared for or in disrepair? Where are street lights located; are they broken, or do they give off adequate light? Are street signs in place? Could strangers find their way around?.

Health Care Climate

To assess the neighborhood's health care climate, students might ask some of the following questions. Is there a neighborhood health facility? How large is it; what area and how many people does it serve? What other health-related services are available in the neighborhood? Students can count the more visible, traditional health care providers: visiting nurse associations, doctors, dentists, chiropractors, optometrists, and podiatrists. Using a map, students can locate themselves and get a feeling for service areas and distances. Where is the nearest hospital? Is this a hospital of choice, or does an individual's health care coverage require the use of another hospital? Students can ascertain if ambulances have easy access to the different parts of the neighborhood.

This is an opportunity to enlarge students' view of health care and health care providers. Do nurse practitioners and nurse midwives practice in the area? Are there psychiatrists or other mental health workers? How would the neighborhood people get this information? Students should consider the role of pharmacists, pharmacies, and medical supplies in health care. Are these services within walking distance of the neighborhood? Is the area safe? Are the hours of operation convenient? Are the neighborhood sidewalks and shopping areas handicap-accessible?

Are there other groups that are concerned about the health and welfare of the neighborhood inhabitants, such as early intervention programs, the Women, Infants, and Children (WIC) nutrition program, hospice programs, or mobile public health programs? In addition, students must consider what part alternative therapies, as well as cultural and indigenous healers, play in providing health care to the people in the neighborhood.

By identifying individuals, groups, and structures that assist individuals with their health care needs, students begin to see the jigsaw puzzle that makes up the health care delivery system. They start to get a sense of how difficult it can be for an individual or family to try to put these pieces together in a meaningful way. This introduction lays the foundation for student involvement with a neighborhood group project.

The initial tour of the neighborhood is an invitation to students to come in and make themselves at home. It is a beginning, a first glimpse. Students' subsequent visits provide opportunities to validate and build on initial impressions, as they continue with observations, data gathering, and reassessments. By helping students tease out and understand the different components that make up a neighborhood, faculty members guide them toward an understanding of the powerful role that environment plays in an individual's health.

LISTENING TO THE NEIGHBORHOOD

The tour of the neighborhood provides the student with an overview of the community. It opens the door and invites the student to come in and meet the people, learn more about its workings and become part of it. In the next step, students meet and talk to the people who make up the neighborhood. These discussions and conversations give the students an appreciation of all the different parts that go into making a whole.

Interacting with Residents

One-to-one contact with neighborhood residents is a valuable part of the process that helps students start to feel included. Involving not only health professionals and community leaders but also selected community residents in the students' orientation provides the opportunity for the students' process of immersion to begin. Residents and students are able to begin a reciprocal process of learning about one another.

Visiting local businesses such as the dry cleaners and the cobblers has led to students' use of these services within the time frame of their clinical day. A drop-off at the start of their clinical time means the work will be completed by the time the students are ready to leave.

Coffee shops and restaurants also provide a social means to meet with residents, experience ethnic foods, and start the development of mutual appreciation. Whether the initial day of a clinical experience includes a buffet luncheon at a local, family-run restaurant or coffee and doughnuts at the deli, students leave feeling more secure in their placement. Comments have included the following: "The food was strange, but the people are interesting"; "They seemed so happy to have us here. I can't wait to come back"; "If Pat can live and raise her family here, it can't be so bad."

Learning from a Spokesperson

The students are also introduced to the concept of the key informant. What sources can they look to provide them with reliable information about the neighborhood? Is there one particular person they should seek out, or are there many? How can the student determine who the best informant would be? After discussing these issues, each student in the group is expected to locate and interview a key informant of his or her choice. There are some general interview guidelines for the student to follow, but they are encouraged to let the informant tell his or her own story (see Appendix C). By regrouping and sharing information, students become aware of the many meanings, needs, and important issues within the same neighborhood.

This exercise is useful in helping students understand that the neighborhood and its residents have their own ideas about what is valuable and important in caring for themselves and others. It is a way to emphasize that faculty and students, as health care providers, are in the neighborhoods in response to requests both explicit and implied, not simply on a "rescue mission" (Freire, 1970).

As the students become more comfortable within their assigned neighborhoods and are able to interact with more people, they begin to realize that "key informant" and "spokesperson" are not synonymous concepts. This fact becomes more obvious when working with different cultural groups. The person who presents him/herself as acculturated to Western ways, manner of dress, English language, abilities, and knowledge of the system is not necessarily the person most trusted by the cultural group to represent its values and best interests. Although it takes time and knowledge of the cultural group in question to come to this realization, it is important to make students aware of this concept from the beginning.

Key informants provide the students with an appreciation of the historical, cultural, and religious beliefs and practices of the neighborhood. By listening to what is said and not said, students come to understand neighborhood concerns. Is it a traditional neighborhood with conservative values? Are group efforts aimed at certain concerns (e.g., food pantries, secondhand clothing drives, bus tours for the elderly, or fund-raising efforts for a drum and bugle corps)? Does the key informant give the impression that the neighborhood is somewhat xenophobic by using terms such as "us" and "them?" Students are encouraged to look for evidence of the neighborhood reaching out to help new groups assimilate, such as the inclusive use of the word "we," and neighborhood functions and groups that seek out and invite participation of the newer inhabitants. Students should come away with some knowledge of neighborhood issues and who defines them. Is the overall impression one of cohesion or divisiveness? If there are multiple issues, is there a sense of common ground from which to work? Is information future-oriented? Is this a neighborhood not only rooted in but also bound to its past, or is it on the move, ready and willing to accommodate to change?

Learning from Individual Residents

Over time, students will interact with more neighborhood inhabitants. Each conversation and observation adds to their knowledge of the workings of the neighborhood. They begin to realize how an individual's or family's religious or cultural beliefs may put them at odds with the dominant culture or system of belief.

Do the people and families they work with feel supported and affirmed within their neighborhood, or is there a "circling of wagons," an us-against-them mentality?

In these situations, faculty members can help students understand that an individual and the neighborhood can approach issues of concern from separate points of view. This does not make one right and the other wrong; rather it makes it imperative that each understand the other's view so that a common ground can be reached and a consensus built that serves all. One example concerns issues of safety, guns, and violence. Violence has become a way of responding to the stresses and frustrations of life. This is especially true in the inner-city neighborhoods. Neighborhood groups, health care professionals included, can no longer look the other way and treat only the aftereffects. Worried neighborhood groups and individuals have issued a cry for increased police protection, gun control, and inclusion of violence prevention into the school curriculum. Teens in the neighborhoods are also concerned. Age-appropriate displays of bravado take on the inappropriate form of owning a gun. This became evident to a group of nursing students on a bus returning home from the neighborhood health center. In the midst of a discussion on neighborhood violence, a teenage high school boy displayed his handgun, indicating his fear for his own safety and his way of handling it. This episode illustrates well how an individual's solution to the problem of safety and violence puts him at odds with the community at large.

With these kinds of observations and experiences, students are helped to understand the larger issues of health care. Maintaining a safe environment is a basic health care concern. In an unsafe environment people are afraid to shop for groceries, fill prescriptions, and exercise and play in the neighborhood. The burden of fear and loss of control add to the everyday stresses of life and increase the physical and social morbidity of the individuals and their neighborhood.

LEARNING NURSING IN THE NEIGHBORHOOD

For learning to take place, it is essential that students feel comfortable in their role and in their neighborhood. To this end, students are encouraged to make use of community services much the same way that an individual from the neighborhood would. By using public transportation, the student begins to appreciate that buses and subway trains are often crowded and not always on time. This leads to an appreciation of what a mother with three children under age 5 must do to get to the health center. It also makes students more empathetic when this mother arrives late for an appointment.

Students visiting the local coffee shops and markets week after week for a meal or a snack get a sense of who some of the neighborhood people are and what their daily lives are like. If someone wants to buy a birthday card, how difficult is that? If some one wants to send a letter or money home to a family in Central or South America, is this service available? If a person needs ostomy care appliances or special foot care dressings, how or where would he or she get it? Are there local programs for infant carseat rentals? This kind of specific information enhances understanding when students plan nursing interventions.

Repeated community assignments over the 3 to 4 years of the clinical nursing components creates an immersion experience into the neighborhood for students. With each return visit, students are able to enter comfortably into a known situation. They greet health center and neighborhood people they know and are welcomed back by people who have been waiting for their return. Because of this level of comfort, students are able to engage in higher level learning activities in more creative and self-directing ways.

NEIGHBORHOOD NEEDS

To begin to identify and meet the neighborhood's health care needs, students are assigned to work with health care providers within the health center and neighborhood. In this way students experience hands-on learning as they work with many different health care professionals and see various health care roles modeled. The neighborhood experience helps students understand and appreciate an enlarged view of health that includes the health of the individual, the health of the group, and the importance of an environment that recognizes risks and diminishes harm.

Such clinical learning experiences may be found within a neighborhood health center and/or other neighborhood settings that include but are not limited to the following:

- Early intervention programs for children
- WIC and other nutritional counseling programs
- Day care centers for infants, toddlers, and children
- Elementary, middle, and high school classroom health education
- School-based clinics, working with the school nurse
- Community and school health fairs
- Outreach programs in mobile health vans, work site clinics, flu clinics
- Governmental programs, such as court systems and housing authorities
- Social service programs, such as food pantries and clothing distribution centers
- Gang projects, battered women's shelter
- Programs for the elderly, such as meal preparation, social clubs and day care
- Support groups of Alcoholics Anonymous and Narcotics Anonymous
- Residential programs such as halfway houses, homeless shelters, mental health residences
- Mental health day programs
- public health nursing.

These activities are described in more depth in Chapters 6 and 7 .

Providing opportunities for students to work with a variety of neighborhood health care providers serves multiple purposes. They become involved in the neighborhood and learn about the people, issues, and values. Working with health care providers also introduces nursing students to the omnipresent and inclusive philosophy of health care that involves a wide range of services. Pre- and postconferences are designed to help students appreciate the idea of health promotion, health education, illness prevention, disease intervention, rehabilitation, and health maintenance. Students begin to sort out the differences and overlaps among nursing care, medical care, surgical care, nutrition services, social services, mental health care, public health, environmental risks, and economic realities about the cost of care and the choices that must be made.

Neighborhood learning experiences help students understand that health care is an integral part of everyday life, that health care is not a service done to or for someone else nor the prerogative of one group of professionals. They learn from their interactions that health is a personal value and individual responsibility based on cultural and family norms. They begin to appreciate the difference between the personal good and the common good and how health care must address both. By using Freire's (1970) model of community empowerment, they understand that meaningful health care agendas are set by the people themselves. They are introduced to the notion that many people and multiple institutions are engaged in the provision of health care services and information. They realize that the role of health care professionals is to use their expert knowledge as facilitators of health care for individuals and neighborhoods, and they become partners with the neighborhood in health care decision making.

SUMMARY

The process of becoming interactive with a neighborhood takes time, but the tone is set and the process begins from the first day the students attend. Involving not only health professionals but also selected community residents, in the students' orientation provides the opportunity for the students' process of immersion to begin. Through key informants and conversations with other residents students are able to establish a valuable base of information from which to provide appropriate health care in this neighborhood. Students' clinical experiences may occur in a neighborhood health center or a wide variety of other sites at which residents congregate within the neighborhood. By having their first clinical experience in nursing take place in the neighborhood, students are introduced to the concept of nursing as occurring wherever the nurse and the client are. The security of the role definition of nursing provided by the institution does not exist. The power differential has changed: the nursing student is a guest in the client's domain. This situation challenges the student to define nursing and nursing care within the context of the caring relationship of nurse, client, family, and community at large.

REFERENCES

Freire, Paulo. (1970). *Pedagogy of the oppressed.* New York: Continuum.
Rubin, H. J., & Rubin, I. S. (1992). *Community organizing and development,* (2nd ed.). New York: Macmillan.
Warren, R. B., & Warren, D. I. (1977). *The neighborhood organizer's handbook.* Notre Dame, Ind.: University of Notre Dame Press.

5

Developing Clinical Activities for Beginning Students

Mary Anne Gauthier

This chapter will give an overview of clinical experiences in the community that are appropriate to BSN students in the first half of their clinical education. In 1978 the World Health Organization recognized that primary health care is the means to attain health care for all. In order to be effective they determined that this care must be practical and scientifically sound, based on socially acceptable methods and technology. For individuals, families, and communities to fully respond to the offer of health care, it must be established with their full participation at a cost in both time and money that can be maintained by the individuals and the community.

Several basic principles of this definition have been incorporated into the neighborhood-based portion of nursing students' clinical experiences as described earlier in this book. First, individuals and communities should be active participants involved in the planning and operation of health care services. Students and nursing faculty enter this arena as potential collaborators with the neighborhood residents and neighborhood health care providers. By returning repeatedly to the same neighborhood, students are able to initiate and then nurture a professional relationship with members of the neighborhood. Second, the provision of health care is only a part of the creation of a healthy neighborhood. Health care providers must also work with individuals in other sectors, such as education, nutrition, agriculture, and housing, to help clients achieve well-being. Basing their works on these principles, nursing faculty members have identified and developed a number of clinical learning experiences, available within neighborhood settings, that enhance the educational development of future nurses.

First, faculty researched local health and demographic trends in the Boston area. According to the Massachusetts Department of Public Health (MDPH), *Health Status Indicators for the Metropolitan Boston Region* (1994), these are broken down into sociodemographic variables, parental and child health, infectious disease, injury, chronic disease, substance abuse, and preventable hospital discharges. Student projects have been developed in conjunction with the neighborhood health centers and community needs assessments. They are designed to individualize the interventions to the targeted needs of the residents and provide a balanced experience for the education of the students. The federal goals of Healthy People 2000 serve as guidelines for health promotion projects and have been a valuable resource to guide teaching about the public health needs of the neighborhoods. Local statistics can be compared to state and national data, and measured against the national goals for improving the health of the population.

To understand the implications of the health status data, the MDPH (1995) provides a variety of data on the residents of the city of Boston as a whole, as well as on various sections. With this data students are able to compare the demographics of the clients in their assigned neighborhood with the city as a whole. Many student projects are developed to target a specific age group, for example, accident prevention programs and safety awareness for school age children and home safety awareness to prevent falls for elders.

Race and ethnicity distribution also effects the way the students' projects are developed. Students learn about the culture and ethnic diversity in the neighborhoods, so language, customs, and norms are incorporated into their care-planning process. In Boston, 58.6% of the residents are white, non-Hispanic; 24.0% are black, non-Hispanic; 10.8% are Hispanic; and 5.1% are Asian (U.S. Census Bureau, 1990). The per capita income is $15,581, which is less than the Massachusetts average of $17,224 (MDPH, 1994). These figures are based on the 1990 census data and reveal that 18.7% of this population have incomes that are less than

100% of the poverty line. The unemployment rate is 6.4% (MDPH, 1994).

These data represent the city of Boston, and the individual neighborhoods vary in age and economic indicators. Nevertheless, these statistics provide some insight into the population with whom the students interact and offer a framework to interpret the potential impacts of the community based curriculum.

UNDERSTANDING THE CONCEPT OF PRIMARY CARE SERVICES

Primary care is the service patients receive at their first point of contact with the health care system (ANA, 1987). It includes health promotion, disease prevention, diagnosis of nursing problems, treatment of selected conditions, and referral to specialty care when required. In the past many nursing education programs have placed more emphasis on preparing nurses for interactions within institutions that provide secondary and tertiary care. Secondary care begins at the point at which specialist and subspecialist services are provided in an office or community hospital inpatient setting. Tertiary care is the level at which highly sophisticated diagnostic, treatment, or rehabilitation services are provided, frequently in university medical centers or equivalent settings (Kelly, 1992). Placed primarily within institutions that provide secondary and tertiary care, nursing students have learned to meet the needs of patients requiring acute or long-term care.

Little has been taught or experienced about the role of nursing in primary care until late in the educational process when a community nursing course generally is offered. As a result, students become well adjusted and acclimated to institutional nursing and then are left with very little time to develop the specialized knowledge base and skills necessary to provide primary care.

Students become comfortable in reacting to a patient's poor health condition but have little or no interest or expertise in providing preventive care to individuals, families, groups, or the community. They tend to look at patients as recipients rather than collaborators in care. With the rapid changes in the health care system, future nurses must not only be able to define primary care but also must be competent and comfortable in the delivery of its services.

EXPLORING THE REALM OF PRIMARY CARE

Primary care providers offer health promotion, preventive care, and continuing care for common health problems and refer clients to specialists when the illness requires more sophisticated care. This definition of primary care goes beyond first contact to include an ongoing coordination of care during health problems and chronic illnesses and emphasizes illness prevention and health maintenance. It recognizes the importance of care over time and across specialty and agency boundaries, as well as the importance of teaching all individuals about health and self-care. With more people living longer, American society is becoming more concerned with health and quality of life. An emphasis on health promotion throughout the life cycle reduces chronic illness and disability in later life.

Examples of settings in which primary care can be delivered include schools, pediatric or family practice clinics, visiting nurse agencies, community health agencies, women's health clinics, meal distribution centers, homeless shelters, courtrooms, camps, group homes, factories, and businesses. In these settings the nurse is usually the first health professional to see the client and has the primary responsibility for monitoring the client.

SKILL DEVELOPMENT IN BEGINNING-LEVEL COURSES

To meet the initial learning needs of students the components of a introductory course concentrate on a core basis of care. The emphasis is on developing nurses capable of delivering health care in community-based settings and fostering consumer responsibility for personal health, self-care, and informed decision making within health care services. Beginning nursing courses generally follow the same pattern of introducing students to technical skills with which they may start to practice. Data collection through interviewing, checking vital signs, and other health assessment skills form the basis of clinical development. Within this new approach the development of basic skills remains; however, the places in which the students learn and practice these skills have changed. Appendix H provides outlines to enhance the development of specific activities at a variety of sites, and student learning experiences in communication, history taking, and health assessment are described below.

Communication

Because a great deal of nursing care involves the use of interpersonal communication skills, the development of these professional skills must be initiated during the first clinical experiences. In community settings opportunities abound for students to develop and enhance their abilities to interview others in a meaningful manner. Individual and group experiences, developed within both casual and formalized structures, allow students to learn from their clients while they develop confidence and increased abilities at their own pace.

To illustrate how communication skills may be fostered, the following example explores students' interactions with adolescents. Nursing students worked to develop an adolescent self-assessment tool to help clinic health providers understand adolescents' needs and provide appropriate services. Students first created an assessment tool based on theoretical premises and then used it to interview the teens. They asked the teens for feedback on the tool. The teens responded quickly that they thought some questions were stupid, such as "What do you watch on TV?" All of the teens agreed that the questions regarding sexual activity, drugs, and smoking were important, but they were not sure the answers would always be truthful. This brought up other questions of what services teens were looking for from nurses and doctors.

History Taking

Students are given various opportunities to interact with community residents and thus develop the skill of dialogue during health history taking. The elderly in particular enjoy working with beginning students. They wait very patiently as the students gingerly move through the process of asking strangers personal questions. Pleased with the attention and proud to be of assistance in the development of students, older people are also generous with their encouragement and praise for the developing student's efforts.

In a neighborhood health center the students learn to introduce themselves to clients and conduct an intake interview, asking the clients why they have come to the clinic and exploring the primary problem. These interviews give the student an opportunity to develop communication skills with a focused objective.

Other students find it helpful to talk with people in the more relaxed atmosphere of the waiting room, on home visits to the elderly, at meal distribution sites, or other gathering places. To focus these conversations the students gather data for an individual cultural assessment (Appendix D) or the development of a health history genogram.

A third type of learning experience incorporates a multidisciplinary aspect by including first-year medical students. A team of three participants, a nursing student, a medical student, and a faculty member, is assigned to interview an elderly person. At the end of the session the participants discuss their experiences. The nursing and medical students also discuss the experience with other members of their clinical groups, exploring their different approaches, analyzing what techniques worked and what did not. During the process the medical and nursing students learn about the differences in their professional focus. Because a faculty member (university- or community-based) is part of each group he or she is able to offer suggestions for future encounters with clients.

Health Assessment

The health assessment of a client involves the assessment of physical and psychological aspects. Health assessment skills are developed from the simple tasks of taking vital signs to the more complex skills of assessing breath sounds and using the otoscope and ophthalmoscope. From the first time they touch a patient to take a pulse to the time when they are able to conduct a basic assessment, students develop most effectively when provided with many opportunities to practice their skills. Within a neighborhood setting students learning nursing skills have access to many opportunities to practice, and as they provide a service to residents, they gain valuable experience through repetitive practice.

Opportunities for developing health assessment skills are available in the health center clinics, day care, and adult day care centers; during blood pressure, hearing, and vision screening programs; and in childhood screening programs in schools.

THEORETICAL CONCEPTS

Theoretical concepts are incorporated and threaded throughout the courses. These concepts are health, culture, collaboration, family, community, and teaching/learning. Each concept is introduced within the didactic and clinical content of each course; however, the students themselves are constantly encouraged to explore how they, their faculty, health care providers, and neighborhood residents define these terms for themselves and how the concepts relate to health care. Their learning experiences are described below.

Health

The more clearly students can define the concept of health, the better able they are to define nursing practice and promote optimal health When interacting with patients, students initially become confused when the patient's definition of health is different from their own. By learning a client's definition, students quickly begin to understand the individualized nature of the concept of optimal health.

To help them explore variations of the definition of health, students conduct surveys that ask residents how they view their own health and what the major health issues are for them, their family, and their community. Students are also assigned to speak to health professionals working in the neighborhood and ask the same questions. In clinical postconference, students share the collective insights that there are many definitions of health and that individuals may view the same state of health differently.

The following examples illustrate the benefits of these experiences. A student was assigned to interview an elderly woman in her home. After the introductions the woman asked if the student could talk with her in her bedroom so that she could sit propped up in bed. The student began the interview with an open-ended question, "How are you doing?" The women answered, "Really good, this is a good day for me."

In postconference the student said that she had accepted the woman's description of how she was. However, what followed amazed her. The woman went on to describe her history of hypertension, her hospitalization for congestive heart failure, her diagnosis of diabetes, and the outcome of an above-the-knee amputation 5 years earlier. She also described the 10 medications she took daily and talked about her family's history of heart disease, hypertension, and diabetes.

When recounting the interview, the student said it was really interesting to talk to someone with this many problems who sees herself as healthy. With assistance from such clients, students come to understand that the way a person defines health is individualistic and determined by many factors.

Students learn best about the factors that influence health behaviors from the clients themselves. For students to be able to work collaboratively with clients, they must have a shared meaning of health. The following interaction between a student and a client demonstrates how a student became enlightened by a client's views of her health and the well-being of her family.

The student interviewed a young mother in the clinic while she was waiting for her appointment. She asked about her health, and the young mother said she was doing well but was really concerned about her new baby. The infant was still in the hospital because she had been delivered at only 2 pounds. The woman talked extensively about how she saw the infant twice a day, pumped her breast milk, and brought it to the hospital. She told the student how she had arranged rides to the hospital for herself each day and laughed when she explained that she had spoken to people in her building whom she had never talked to before to ask for rides because it was so important to her to see her baby, provide the breast milk, and hold her. The student was impressed with the woman's sense of being a mother.

The student and client then entered the clinic area to see the nurse. The woman, who lived near the clinic, was coming in daily to have her cesarean section dressing changed and healing process assessed. All the time the dressing was being changed, the women spoke only of the baby, her eagerness to get to the hospital, to hold the baby, to bring the breast milk. As the incision was exposed, packed, and redressed, the student was shocked to see a wound 6 inches by 2 inches. Yet the woman reported that she was "fine." "Did you have any pain?" "No." "Are you tired?" "Yes, but it's because I didn't sleep. I was worried about getting to the hospital on Saturday, and then when I was getting the mail today, I asked a neighbor who had a car if he would take me on Saturday and he said yes. I'll take a nap this afternoon."

In response to the mother's need for transportation the nurse investigated and located a source of taxi vouchers. This intervention removed the concern and the time consumed in arranging transportation. The mother could then focus on resting in preparation for the eventual homecoming of her infant. The student was amazed at how the woman viewed her health condition and that transportation to see her infant was more important to her than rest.

From this experience the student learned the woman's definition of health. She practiced her interviewing skills and had the opportunity to watch a professional nurse care for a client in a holistic manner. Beyond the care of the incision, the nurse supported the woman's goals to maintain daily contact with her baby and to breast-feed; she encouraged the woman's mothering by praising her resourcefulness and determination. The importance of focusing on more than wound care became apparent to the student. A secondary gain was that the student was able to observe the process of wound assessment and care in the context of a holistic primary care situation.

Culture

The concept of cultural differences may be addressed in class in relation to any number of health practices (e.g., nutrition, child care practices, medication use). This information is interesting yet limited in effect when a student tries to develop a plan of care with an individual of a specific culture. Students not only must understand that different cultures have different beliefs, they must also learn how to determine an individual's cultural beliefs and how they will affect the current situation. Students learn from their clients by conducting cultural assessments (refer to Appendix D) and participating in forums developed and conducted by community residents to explore and teach about variations between and among people of different cultures. Right from the beginning, students are sensitized to the fact that recipients may view health care services from a framework that is different from the student's. Students learn about cultural barriers that obstruct care and how to attempt to bridge the gap.

During client encounters students are encouraged to recognize then put aside their assumptions and to learn from their client. When conducting nutritional assessments before diet teaching, students learn that different cultures have meal patterns different from their own. For example, when listing the foods she had eaten during the past 24 hours, a Haitian woman described each meal. The student related later, "It sounded like her day was mixed up. She started the day with a meal we would call dinner, and her last meal was what we could call breakfast." With cultural sensitivity the student was able to support this pattern of eating while continuing to assess the woman's overall nutritional intake.

Collaboration

Although health professionals work side by side and in teams, they do not always understand one another's expertise or consider the attainment of common goals. Collaboration between professionals facilitates effective client care by encouraging information sharing, comprehensive planning, and continuity of care. Within the neighborhood setting the collaborative health care team considers the client as a central member of the team. A collaborative relationship, which promotes joint problem solving, develops when each member of the health team recognizes and accepts the unique contribution made by others.

Students are asked to identify members of the health team, their role with the client, and the unique role of nursing. Students interview members of the health team and ask how they perceive their roles. They also learn the varying amounts of preparation for practice, educational diversity, and the credentials necessary for each member of the team.

A student noted in her log that in practice there is a blur be-

tween the roles of the health care team—professionals and support staff. The professionals have completed a program and
passed a licensing exam. The support staff consists of individuals
such as clerical workers and laboratory technicians who assist
professionals in the delivery of health care. But sometimes the activities are interchanged, as when the professional draws the
blood work and the support staff asks the client the reason for
the clinic visit.

Family

Family has been defined in the literature in a number of different
ways. Students learn about the definition of family from the residents themselves when they are paired with resident families interested in sharing their life experiences. Over time the family includes the student in its life experiences, especially health care
concerns, as members become acutely or chronically ill and families grow or decrease in size.

To initiate this learning experience the health center asks for volunteers from its clientele. The center hosts a luncheon at which each
student meets representatives from the volunteer family. Over time
the student makes home visits and meets with a family member at
least three times in each course or when he or she seeks care at the
health center. In some cases the student may also continue the relationship through telephone contact. The purpose of these meetings
is for the student to learn from the family member(s) about their
health-related needs and then assist the family as needed in meeting those needs. Each student-family relationship develops at a different pace and in a different manner. Some dyads continue in close
relationship over the years of clinical education. Others grow apart
as the interests and needs of the family members and the students
diverge. Whether or not the experience is long-lived, the students
learn about reality from the interaction. The family members express
a sense of raised self-esteem that they are valuable teachers to the
developing health professionals.

Community

Two of the goals of basing undergraduate education in the community are to help students understand people as they live in

their community and to enable students to deliver nursing care where the people live, work, and go to school. Several projects were designed to meet this goal.

Learning activities, such as the Environmental Survey (Appendix E) and the Interview with Key Informant (Appendix C), allow students to polish their observation and interviewing skills while becoming more familiar with the community. Tours led by residents of the neighborhood, lunch in a local restaurant, and visits to the library, churches, courts, and other community settings all help students understand how the community is experienced by those who live there.

Learning about a neighborhood and its residents begins with students' first clinical experience and continues throughout the remainder of their educational experience. The process continues because the students return to the same neighborhood for clinical experience for the duration of their clinical education.

Client Teaching/Learning

Differences in client population and the delivery of health care make meeting clients' needs for health education not only more critical but also more challenging. The teaching and learning project is a special part of the beginning community experience for nursing students. The purpose of each project is to have the student, in collaboration with others, plan, develop, implement, and evaluate a health promotion project. To meet these challenges, students need knowledge and skills relevant to teaching and effective learning.

All proposals grow out of interactions with community providers and residents. They are based in the reality of the needs of the residents and developed after research within the community. Students investigate the need and potential effect of preventive interventions. At the same time they learn that to be successful a health care intervention must agree with the priorities of the client, whether individual, family, group, or community. Students then develop a proposal before proceeding with the development of their project (see Appendix F).

As part of the process students create a project budget. They are asked to consider financial as well as time expenditures. Students are very creative and have discovered many resources, such as supplies, pamphlets, and models, available in the neighborhood, from state and local health departments, and from nonprofit organizations, to support their health promotion projects.

Before a teaching projects is carried out, it is reviewed and discussed in clinical conference. This allows the students to obtain feedback from their peers and instructor, and it helps reinforce the fact that the student is capable and has the knowledge to carry out the project.

STUDENTS EXPERIENCES PROVIDING CARE WITHIN A NEIGHBORHOOD

Primary care nursing is oriented to health promotion, disease prevention, the diagnosis nursing problems, and referral when required. A goal of primary care is to improve the level of health through preventive health services, environmental protection, and health education. Health promotion activities enhance well-being, whereas disease prevention activities protect persons from disease and its consequences. There are three levels of prevention: primary, secondary, and tertiary. Nursing care activities developed and implemented by students during their beginning clinical courses have occurred at all three levels, with a particular focus on meeting the health care needs of individuals, families, and groups.

Primary Prevention

Primary prevention is the prevention of health problems before they occur. Primary prevention includes health education programs, immunizations, and physical and nutritional activities. It occurs before the development of disease or dysfunction and focuses on decreasing the probability of a specific illness or dysfunction occurring. The recipients of care are considered physically and emotionally healthy and may be an individual, family, group, or community.

Individual

Three students spent 2 days in a preschool day care center and observed 3- and 4-year-old children playing and socializing with each other. They were there from the time the children came in the morning through the play period, snack, story time, and preparation for lunch. The students observed the children's personal hygiene (using the bathroom, washing their hands, sneezing) and proposed to the teacher that they develop a program related to this area. They wrote goals and a plan, which they discussed with their instructor and the day care teacher. They researched age-appropriate teaching for this age group. Then they obtained toothbrushes and toothpaste from local dental offices and produced a poster of a great tooth monster that showed what happened to unbrushed teeth. They demonstrated and had the children brush their teeth with toothbrushes. They also set up a rack where the children could leave their toothbrushes each day and commended the staff members for their willingness to include toothbrushing in the children's day.

Later, one of the students wrote in her journal: "I learned a lot about small children yesterday. I've never been with little kids much. I didn't realize how hard it was to keep their attention and that their attention span was so short. I'm really glad I had this opportunity to spend time with the kids and to also help them. I'm surprised that I really feel like I accomplished something. I didn't expect to feel this way."

Other students used the medium of finger painting to teach the children about hand washing. The nursing students invited the children to play with finger paints. However, they adjusted the time allotment so that the emphasis was shifted to cleaning their hands rather than painting. In groups of three or four the children came to the water table to wash the paint off their hands. This was a new activity for them because the teachers usually washed their hands for them. With instruction and encouragement the young children derived a great deal of pleasure in cleaning their hands themselves.

Returning to the classroom during the following 2 weeks the nursing students assessed whether the students were still attempting to wash their own hands. They reinforced the original lesson, this time using soap, and praised the children as they attempted to follow this health practice.

With a slightly older group of clients the importance of handwashing was reinforced by having the children make agar prints of their hands. A week later they were shown how many microbes had grown.

Family

After working in the pediatric clinic, a nursing student, through talking to the physician, nurses, staff, and parents in the waiting room, became aware of the high number of accidents among toddlers. She discussed with her instructor and the clinical coordinator a possible project on home safety. Her primary objective was to raise parental awareness of the dangers present in all houses. She made a poster that showed every room in the house and the potential dangers to small children. She then sat in the waiting room and talked to parents, using the poster as a guide. As a sophomore student she was surprised at the reception she received from the parents and acknowledged that she felt comfortable in this situation. The poster hangs in the clinic today as a visible reminder of the student project and continues to educate parents on safety issues.

Group

A nursing student in a elderly meal distribution site attended a blood pressure screening program with the seniors. While at the site she sat with a group of seniors and asked what type of health information they were interested in. At first the seniors were vague about their interests. Gradually, they began to talk and ask questions about high cholesterol, low cholesterol, "good" lipids, "bad" lipids, and diet. They talked with the students about food labeling and what that meant. After the students spent time with the elderly, they discussed their ideas and what they thought the concerns of the elderly were in relation to diet. The students went back to the elder group and verified that cholesterol, fats, and labeling were concerns of the elders. Together they decided what information they would present. The students gathered information about cholesterol, fats, and food labels. They made posters and handouts. The following is a quote from the student's journal after the session: "I'm really surprised at how much I knew about cholesterol. It was fun to tell someone else and to know they were really interested. I didn't think I could talk to a group before this. Once I got started, I felt really good. I think they liked it too."

Such an experience offered a chance to assess older adults in a well setting. The students became aware of the vision and hearing deficits of the elderly and the need to adjust their speaking and written material accordingly. They learned that these elderly people lived at home independently and would use this information when they went shopping and in cooking. They learned that the elderly are continuing to learn, interested in keeping up to date, and willing to change eating habits if given a good reason.

Another student developed a health prevention intervention for a different group of clients. She worked with a group of special-needs teens regarding the basic food groups and good nutrition. After giving the children information about the food pyramid, she gave them pictures cut from magazines to paste on a poster. It surprised the nursing student that she could involve the children in the project and teach them about good nutrition.

The student noted later, "In this experience I had a chance to challenge myself with something that I thought was impossible, was totally different from anything I expected to do in nursing, and beyond my imagination a few months ago. I never thought I could teach. I never thought I would work with special needs children. I'm glad I had the chance."

Community

Illegal drug use, the prevention of AIDS transmission, and violence are three areas of concern to community residents that students have addressed.

The use of illegal drugs is a problem in many communities. To address this issue nursing and medical students researched the literature regarding effective drug education and talked to children in the elementary, middle school, and junior high grades. The students then involved the children in developing a booklet to teach their peers not to use drugs. Once completed, the booklet was translated into the six languages used in the community. Now the booklet is used by other students when they work with school-age children and is available to the schools for use.

Transmission of the AIDs virus is a problem within many communities. To decrease the risk, condom use is suggested. Developing a prevention program based on condom use requires the assistance of neighborhood residents. A nursing student, working very closely with a community educator, developed a program to recruit neighborhood women as consultants in the project. At the resulting meeting examples of several programs tried in other communities were presented. The community residents selected the program they felt would work best in their community. They selected a process of small gatherings or parties, much like "Tupperware parties," at which a trained resident teaches the guests about the transmission of the virus. Concerns about how to obtain condoms and how to ensure that a sexual partner uses them were also addressed. The program has been extremely successful because the neighborhood consultants used their knowledge to select a culturally acceptable format; they determined what terms for body parts and sexual intercourse could be used without being offensive, and publicized the program to their friends. The student provided the resources, and the residents provided the knowledge of what was acceptable.

A third example addresses the concern of violence. A nursing student was invited to attend a meeting of community leaders to address an urgent concern about violence prevention. The attendees—five clergy and two community leaders, a health care provider, and the nursing student—gathered in response to the news that a well-known sneaker manufacturer was close to releasing a new line of basketball sneakers labeled "Run and Gun." The student reported back at postconference that at first she didn't understand what this activity had to do with nursing. As the meeting progressed, she found that her knowledge about human growth and development and a concern about the health and well-being of her clients led to her becoming very involved in the discussion about what, if anything, should be done. A request to the corporate lawyers to change the name was rejected because of the cost already involved in product development. The group then drew on its collective resources and prepared statements to be distributed through various religious denominations asking for a boycott of the company. The corporate lawyers were notified of this action, and a week later the name of the sneaker was changed to "Run and Slam," which carries a less violent connotation. The student related amazement at the power of a few people to make such a significant statement, altering the potential for health and safety within this and other neighborhoods.

Secondary Prevention

Secondary prevention is care aimed at early recognition and treatment of disease. It includes general nursing interventions and teaching early signs of disease conditions, plus care activities such as screening and diagnosis and treatment of health problems. Screening, an essential element, involves assessment of particular groups of people for specific illness.

Individual

Two students recognized that when a new mother called the clinic because her baby was sick, one of the first pieces of information they needed was the infant's temperature. Assessment of a new mother's knowledge about temperature taking was incorporated into their care process. When the mother was unsure or uncomfortable about the procedure, they taught her how to use and read a thermometer and when to call the clinic.

Students work with the nurse in the health center clinic conducting nurse visits. One interaction was with a client there for an evaluation of her activity level and diet and to have her blood sugar tested. The nurse knew the client from weekly visits and ongoing teaching sessions. The student was included as a provider within the session and learned about the needs of a diabetic patient from the client and also the value of a long-term relationship.

Family

A student was assigned to work with an older women visiting the clinic to receive nutrition counseling for the treatment of her hypertension. He explained to the woman and her adult son, with whom she lived, that both could benefit from adopting the same dietary program. He explored with them their current dietary habits and suggested ways to make appropriate adjustments that were also culturally and economically feasible. At the conclusion of the session the student was encouraged by the positive response of the mother and son and believed that because the dietary changes were being incorporated into the life-style of the cohabitants they had a better chance of being maintained. The student was pleased with the possibility that his intervention could affect not just one person but all members of the household.

Group

Hearing loss, which is common in the elderly, can lead to withdrawal from social contact, with resulting isolation and depression. A common cause of hearing loss is cerumen buildup in the ears. Students established a hearing screening program at a day care site for the elderly. They screened the participants' hearing and checked for cerumen buildup. When difficulties were identified, clients were referred to the clinic for wax removal and follow-up if hearing aids were required.

Other students conducted a blood pressure screening and education program at a housing site for the elderly. During the process they encountered an unexpected problem with the vision of many clients. The students said, "One problem was the inability of the clients to read the handouts on blood pressure because of poor eyesight. We tried to overcome this by reviewing the information with them and then suggesting they ask relatives or people they were living with to read it to them." Further evaluation of the process demonstrated that the students learned more from this experience than how to take blood pressures. "It would have been better to recognize the potential for this vision problem earlier. If we had anticipated it, we could have allowed for more time to be spent with each person to talk and to go over the handouts," one student said.

Tertiary Prevention

Tertiary prevention nursing care is carried out with patients with chronic diseases. Activities include patient instruction on how to manage these diseases. Parkinson's disease, diabetes, and multiple sclerosis lend themselves to tertiary prevention. The goals as to prevent further deterioration of physical and mental functions, and to help patients utilize whatever residual function is available for maximum quality of life. Rehabilitation is an essential part of tertiary prevention. This type of nursing care recognizes that a health problem cannot always be cured but can be stabilized. It can help a person adjust to that disease. Tertiary prevention focuses on helping a person live with the condition and meet the demands of daily living while preventing further complications

Individual

A nursing student in an adult day care setting taught an overweight 83–year-old woman with hypertension and a history of constipation, arthritis, and immobility the benefits of increasing the fiber in her diet. She taught her to identify foods containing fiber and to recognize the recommended serving size of the fiber-rich foods.

Group

The school nurse identified 30 children in a middle school (fourth, fifth, and sixth graders), out of a school population of 600, who had asthma and were currently using inhalers in school. Two nursing students developed an educational program explaining the condition of asthma and its treatment, not only for the children with asthma but also for their classmates. The first part of the program described asthma, using lectures, drawings, pictures, and handouts. The nursing students created an atmosphere in which afflicted and nonafflicted children could ask questions. The nursing students were impressed with the afflicted children's understanding of their condition and the effects of stress, diet, and activity on their condition. When nonasthmatic children asked questions, the asthmatic children often hopped in to answer before the nursing students had an opportunity to do so.

The second part of the program explained the different types of inhalers and medicines used by afflicted students. Again both groups of students asked many questions. Students were taught about how the medication content differed from one inhaler to another. There was much discussion about different treatment regimens and why one child could not use another's inhaler. The participants in the program learned about the condition of asthma and its treatment. The nonafflicted children understood better the health situation the asthmatic children were dealing with on a daily basis.

This program introduced the nursing student to middle-school age children who are well except for asthma. They learned about the various levels of development among children of the same and slightly different ages. The teachers who attended saw the nursing students as the experts and asked them questions. One of the nursing students was a respiratory therapist and had more extensive knowledge of asthma than most beginning nursing students have. This topic allowed him to use his past experiences not only to teach the schoolchildren but also his peers, instructor, school nurse, and schoolteachers. While providing this teaching intervention, the students, both male and female, served as role models for children considering careers in the health professions. Interested students asked questions about choosing these careers.

A less direct care interaction also provided a service to a group of individuals at risk. A student telephoned all the high-risk clients to remind them to come to the clinic for their flu shot. The list was prepared by the clinic's nurse and doctor. The student prepared a script about the date of the flu clinic and the reasons these client should attend. Most likely as a result of this interaction, 80% of the clients called by the student came to the clinic for a flu shot. Although the student was not part of the actual administration of the vaccine, she played an important role in the health of the clients.

A group of special-needs students were surveyed about their interest in a particular health issue. They decided on "how to keep their skin looking good." The nursing students prepared a program about personal hygiene and grooming for the students. In the process, the nursing students learned that special-needs teenagers are interested in the opposite sex and concerned about their appearance.

In adult day care settings students help the elderly with personal hygiene. Atherosclerosis, diabetes, and other circulation problems found in the aged can cause small cuts, hangnails, calluses, and ulcers to develop into serious health care problems. Students in adult day care services have the opportunity to examine feet, nails, shoes, canes, crutches, and prosthetics. They assess for correctly fitting shoes, the presence of skin breakdown, and irritation. During the evaluation process they teach the basics of good foot care.

SUMMARY

Primary care is an essential but often under represented area in nursing education. The role of the nurse in primary, secondary, and tertiary prevention is a vital component in addressing the health care needs of individuals, families, groups, and the community. Within a neighborhood setting there are many opportunities for beginning nursing students to develop professional nursing skills while simultaneously addressing issues of diversity in health beliefs, cultural diversity, family, and the roles of members of the multidisciplinary care team.

REFERENCES

American Nurses Association. (1987). *Position statement on primary care.* Washington, DC: Author.

Kelly, L. (1992). *Dimensions of professional nursing.* New York: Macmillan.

Massachusetts Department of Public Health. (1995). *Health status indicators: Community health network areas, Metro Boston region.* Boston, MA: MDPH.

U.S. Census Bureau. (1990).

World Health Organization. (1978). *Definition of Health.* Geneva: Author.

6

Developing Clinical Activities for Advanced Students

Margaret Ann Mahoney

Within a community-based curriculum, the knowledge, skills, and attitudes necessary for nursing practice continue to be developed across all the nursing courses. As students progress through the curriculum, they return to the same neighborhood for clinical practicum time. Clinical experiences designed for learning the nursing concentrations of mental health, reproductive and developmental health, and medical/surgical and rehabilitation care each contain a community component. As students acquire increasing confidence and skills in communication, critical thinking, and nursing therapeutics, they are able to assume a more independent role in providing care within neighborhood sites. During one of their final clinical courses, community health, the students have the opportunity to demonstrate synthesis of their knowledge by designing and implementing an aggregate experience for their clinical neighborhood. During this course they focus on the public health needs of a group of people in the community and operationalize the concepts of primary health care that they have learned.

LEARNING WITH A COMMUNITY INSTRUCTOR

During the first clinical year, the students were introduced to the health care providers and community leaders in each neighborhood health center. As they advance in the nursing program, the students develop collaborative relationships with these health care providers and neighborhood leaders during their clinical time. In their junior and senior years the students move to an educational model in which they collaborate more closely with community instructors. Students, community instructors, and university faculty plan clinical experiences that will meet the objectives of each course. Each student signs a contract for a particular educational experience with a community instructor, who will work with the student during clinical time under the guidance and direction of the college of nursing faculty. These instructors may be community nurses in a variety of roles: in the neighborhood schools, rehabilitation residences or group homes, or homeless shelters. Students also may contract with instructors from other disciplines, such as mental health or outreach workers, victim witness advocates in the courts, childbirth educators, coordinators of programs for immigrants, or peer support networks such as groups for substance abusers or family caregivers. An example of this student/community instructor contract appears in Appendix G.

Within this framework students have the choice to explore a variety of interests or to concentrate on working with a particular population group or site of care. Some students choose a population group, such as people with HIV. In initial clinical courses they may accompany an outreach worker or a driver who delivers hot meals and gain interview skills and home visiting experience. They begin to interact with clients in delivery of support services, and as they gain nursing experience, they can continue to make home visits to provide more skilled care. Initially, the students are closely supervised; however, as their expertise grows, they are able to develop a care plan and implement nursing interventions with a greater degree of autonomy.

The students who choose to work with a selected population are able to investigate the network of community agencies involved in meeting the health care needs of that particular group. They learn about the range of services from peer support groups to hospice care. Providers include students in planning meetings, community programs, and training sessions for professional development seminars so that students are able to learn about the full scope of care available to their selected population. With their community instructors and nursing faculty, they determine where their developing nursing skills might be needed. For example, if they choose to focus on the problems of families with HIV-infected children, the community offers a broad array of opportunities that meet the objectives of each nursing specialty course and expand the student's awareness of the implications of this disease.

In their initial health teaching the students may address an elementary school class on the body changes they will experience with pubescence, a junior high school class on making health-affirming choices to avoid alcohol and drugs, or a high school class on the dangers of sexually transmitted diseases, especially HIV. When these students study maternal and child health, they may teach parenting skills or provide care for mothers and children who are HIV-positive in one of the shelters or group homes. During their mental health course, the students may become involved in family support groups or become part of a hospice team. By the senior year the student has acquired the knowledge of community resources necessary for a case management role and a truly holistic perspective. Appendix I provides outlines that further explain the development of some activities.

COMMUNICATION

The oral and written communication skills of students are expanded through community clinical placements. The emphasis on interview and assessment continues throughout the curriculum, with the students taking a more active role in developing and implementing nursing care plans as their own knowledge of nursing increases. They have many opportunities to share this knowledge of health care with others across the life span. Students are expected to plan and implement age-appropriate and culturally sensitive presentations and programs for diverse audiences, from preschoolers to the elderly. They become adept at communicating health promotion concepts, and through their active involvement in developing and presenting programs, they learn about the importance of being role models for healthy life-styles for the residents of the neighborhood.

Primary Prevention

As discussed in the previous chapter, primary prevention is heath care that occurs before the development of disease or dysfunction. The focus is on decreasing the probability of a specific illness or dysfunction occurring in an otherwise healthy individual, family, group, or community. One example of a student initiated program in primary prevention is home visits for safety evaluations. The elders who attend day programs run by the Councils on Aging are introduced to the students, who interview them as part of their health assessments. For those who consent, the students and outreach workers make home visits and inspect the homes for potential hazards. Scatter rugs, overloaded electrical outlets, and loose rails and bannisters are hazardous for elders. Emergency response systems, grab rails in bathrooms, and arrangements for minor home repairs can make the home environment safer for elderly residents and prevent falls and injuries. The Councils on Aging have developed a home safety evaluation checklist that the students can use, and referral sources are available to remedy the problems they identify. Sometimes the students have enlisted other family members in these home projects. Students have become more aware of adaptations that can be made for elders who wish to remain independent in spite of physical limitations. When they are in hospital clinical settings, they use this knowledge in their discharge planning and ask detailed questions about the home environment. They know how to obtain community services based on their assessments of the elders' ability to function safely at home.

Secondary Prevention

Secondary prevention includes the early recognition and treatment of illness. In one situation the students' communication skills were evident after a chemical spill forced the closing of a day care center and an elementary school. Four hundred families in the neighborhood were affected, and the community voiced concerns about potential health risks from exposure to these chemicals. The nursing students obtained information about the hazardous materials from the state and prepared informational flyers in simple language for parents of the children. They also organized a community meeting to address the residents' concerns. To advertise the event students made flyers and obtained the services of a translator for the handouts and the event. Fortunately, the potential hazards were not serious, and the community members stated that they understood the situation much better and felt their needs for information and reassurance were met by this student activity. Because they were familiar with the neighborhood and participated in the activities of the health center, the students were able to mobilize quickly to respond to this potential public health crisis and address the residents' fears appropriately.

Tertiary Prevention

The knowledge of community resources that the students acquire is freely shared with patients and hospital providers. The students do a lot of health education in the community, and their knowledge of resources and communication skills enhance their patient teaching. In the advanced nursing courses, the faculty begin to see that, because the students spend clinical time in both hospitals and communities, their knowledge is carried across practice sites. For example, during the hospital maternity rotation, in which inpatient stays are brief, students were teaching new mothers about community programs, such as supplemental nutrition for women, infants, and children (the WIC program), which provides food stamps and nutrition counseling for this population. The students were able to match the needs of the patients to the income eligibility guidelines and make appropriate referrals so that services could begin at discharge. The staff nurses were so impressed that they asked the clinical instructor if the students could provide them with an in-service education program to update their knowledge of these community programs. The students were happy to oblige and left a resource book with pamphlets and information that the staff nurses could use. One student wrote that the self-esteem of her group was given quite a boost when the staff nurses asked them for information, as usually it was the other way around.

CULTURE

Cultural sensitivity awareness begins with an understanding of one's own cultural beliefs and of the process of socialization into a health care profession. Interdisciplinary seminars are held each term, so an understanding of these values and beliefs extends across health professions. There is a traditional culture of medicine that differs from the profession of nursing. The students from each discipline begin to appreciate each other through sensitivity workshops in which they are asked to develop a list of adjectives describing physicians, nurses, and social workers. These papers are collected. Next, each student interviews a student from a different discipline and writes a new list that describes the person he or she interviewed. As a third step, students pair up and interview a health care professional, again making a list of adjectives that describe this person. These lists are then compared and discussed in a seminar. The similarities, strengths, and stereotypes are examined in context of their experience of each other. The students learn a great deal about their own values and beliefs and about other disciplines. They can then apply this knowledge about presumptive biases to their self-critique when interacting with other cultures and ethnic groups.

Because a great deal of time and effort is spent on sensitizing students to the diverse cultures encountered in the city, students are very aware of the importance of respecting the client's individuality, values, and beliefs. The census data do not adequately discriminate among the Caribbean, Latin American, and African cultures that can be found within the city. Also, each of these categories, encompasses many diverse groups. The students learn not to stereotype a community resident based on appearance or these broad categories, but to make meaningful distinctions, for example, between a native African-American, a Haitian who speaks Creole, and a Cape Verdean who speaks Portuguese. They are able to individualize their care plans to include the patients' cultural values and beliefs and to specify the need for a translator if necessary. Health teaching about diet, exercise, stress reduction, risk behaviors, and environmental or occupational hazards are client-centered and culturally sensitive. The students learn about the folk healers and family remedies that are used to treat illnesses and incorporate that knowledge into their interventions. They visit the local pharmacists and the health food and specialty markets to inquire about alternative treatments. As a result of these experiences, one student identified a woman who was giving her infant a prescription medication for an ear infection and at the same time an herbal preparation that contained a controlled substance. She was able to correctly assess the baby's lethargy as the result of a drug overdose from the combined effect of the prescribed medication and the folk treatments. Dose adjustments were made, and the child improved. Based on her research, the health center staff became aware of a local supplier of home remedies that could cause drug reactions. As more immigrants arrive in our city, this cultural awareness of health care beliefs and folk practices must be incorporated into the students' curriculum and our health care teaching.

Primary Prevention

The majority of the students are young adults, recently emerged from the adolescent years. Adolescence is a culture they believe they know well, and they are able to relate to the developmental needs and pressures of this age group. Adolescent pregnancy is a problem in the city, and 4.8% of births in 1992 ($n = 444$) were to teen mothers under age 18 (MDPH, 1994). Many of the students have collaborated with neighborhood providers to focus on building the self-esteem of the teens and work with various youth groups to prevent teen pregnancy. Several groups of students worked with teens to produce videos aimed at building self-esteem. Together, in weekly meetings during the term, they wrote rap songs, choreographed dances, and produced these films. They showed them to other teens in school assemblies and community meetings. These videos were then donated to the neighborhood health centers, where they are played in the clinic waiting rooms.

Secondary Prevention

In Boston the high school dropout rate is one of the worst in the state. This fact, combined with an increase in immigration, means that there are a great number of functionally illiterate and non-English speaking residents of the neighborhoods. The nursing students have spent clinical time in classes for English as a second language (ESL) and high school equivalency (GED). They have presented seminars about the services available at the neighborhood health centers and the importance of immunizations and have conducted screenings for hypertension and tuberculosis. Some students who are able to speak a second language have become more involved with the classes and have conducted prenatal and parenting skills workshops.

Because the incidence of breast cancer is less common in Asian women, this screening practice is not taught routinely. However, after the women emigrate to the United States and adopt some of our habits, their incidence of breast cancer increases. To address this increased risk the women were taught the techniques of self-examination after their English classes. Many of the women brought their husbands, and several of the male members of the classes also attended. The translators in the health center assisted the student to prepare handouts for the class and helped with the presentation. These materials are now available to the health center staff for teaching Vietnamese women about breast self-examination.

Tertiary Prevention

In the neighborhoods the students learned about the impact of violence on residents. Data collected in 1992 indicated that the rate of homicide deaths was 12.2 per 100,000 residents in the city of Boston. This compares with an overall state rate of 3.9 and a national rate of 10.4 (MDPH, 1994). Children all know relatives or friends who have been wounded or killed, and elders are afraid to leave their homes. Some students have provided clinical care for clients who later met a violent death. Others developed a personal involvement by caring for clients during the restorative process.

In response to the community-identified need and their own interactions, many students wanted to become active in solutions. Working with community members, the students became involved in conflict resolution workshops, educated providers about safe houses for women, worked directly with victims of domestic violence within shelters, and participated in the development and implementation of a gun buy-back program. In one summer semester more than 200 weapons were turned in, and the students felt very positive about their contribution to decreasing the spread of violence in the city.

One group of students conducted a grief workshop in an elementary school. The film by Leo Buscaglia titled *Freddy the Leaf* discusses death as part of the changing seasons in the life of one leaf. The boys and girls were attentive during the film and afterward shared their stories of loss of pets, friends, and relatives. The nursing students identified those youngsters who had sustained losses and assessed their support systems and coping ability. They spent time with these children, observing them in classes and during playtime, and made referrals to the school nurse and guidance department for those students who needed more skilled services or further support. Students also had the opportunity to work with professional play therapists and to observe children who are victims of family violence through one-way mirrors. They then stayed with the children while their parents went in for formal counseling and group sessions. These experiences helped them assess children at school who may be acting out due to their experiences with violence at home or in their communities.

The nursing students, who are often from suburban or rural areas, expressed amazement at the children's firsthand knowledge of violence. They also were impressed by the children's willingness to share their stories and by how articulate and attentive they were. Through their work in the elementary school the nursing students gained a deeper understanding of the role of the school system in health promotion and the effect of home and community violence on our youth.

Other students had the opportunity to observe police department personnel respond to 911 calls. As they sat with the emergency operator and monitored calls for a session, they became aware of the problems faced by first responders. They learned about the types of calls that come into the 911 system and the triage skills used on the telephone to respond appropriately. This interdisciplinary experience will enhance the students' appreciation for the skills of emergency personnel and understanding of how community resources are deployed in a crisis situation. This interaction also exposed students to the experience of recipients of these services and may foster greater collaboration when students work in emergency settings of tertiary care facilities.

COLLABORATION

As the above example illustrates, interdisciplinary collaboration is an important part of this community-based primary care curriculum. Students learn about health care from all members of the health care team and from community residents as well. When faculty collaborate with community residents and health center providers to plan, implement, and evaluate the clinical experiences for students, they serve as role models of collaborative practice for the students.

Primary Prevention

All students participate in health fairs. At first, students participate by preparing and presenting informational booths about nutrition, exercise, and safety awareness. As their expertise increases, they participate more actively in the overall development and implementation of health fairs. The upper-division students have organized and run health fairs for schools, workplaces, and elder care sites independently by making contacts with community leaders they have met and worked with in earlier rotations. The students have conducted these events in schools, the community college, the YMCA, and adult day health care centers. They have involved the teachers, guidance counselors, physical and occupational therapists, dentists, medical students, nutritionists, and mental health professionals. They have also collaborated with other organizations, such as the American Cancer Society, the American Heart Association, and the Alzheimer's Association. Graduate practitioner students have participated in these fairs, providing screening and primary care services. These activities have brought various community groups together, promoting not only the health of the neighborhoods but also opportunities for further collaboration.

Secondary Prevention

As students progress in the program, they enjoy practicing their newly acquired skills. Flu clinics are very popular with the students because they provide experiences with administration of injections. Students also conduct tuberculosis, diabetes, and cholesterol screenings in the community and vision, hearing, and scoliosis testing with school nurses. When organizing these screenings, the students learn about the process of informed consent and the necessary provision of follow up services. They have worked with the medical students and health center staff when referrals are needed.

They have translated standard forms into the primary languages of the neighborhoods or enlarged the print for health screenings in elder care sites. Each of these efforts adds to the materials that the neighborhood health centers have available to improve access to their health care services.

Tertiary Prevention

Students have enjoyed clinical experiences in the early intervention programs for infants and toddlers with disabilities and have been part of core evaluations for school age children. Teachers, therapists, and social workers have welcomed their input, and students have gained an understanding of the process of multidisciplinary collaboration for children with multiple needs. By learning of the contributions made by other members of the team, they become more aware of the role of the nurse. They are able to contribute their knowledge to the care plan and know when to make referrals. They are able to center on the needs of the client and gain holistic insights into the process of planning to meet care needs. Nursing students attend the interdisciplinary conferences and are given a series of questions to consider about the roles of the team members, the goals of the meeting, and the development of the interdisciplinary plan of care. These are discussed in clinical conference, with the medical and nursing student groups together.

FAMILY

Because students begin to make home visits in the first year and remain with the same neighborhood, they learn about health care problems and disease in the context of the family. Acute and chronic illness are encountered, and the impact on the family is always assessed. The students learn to enlist family members as care providers and how to negotiate care plans according to family wishes.

Primary Prevention

Teen pregnancy is a problem of increasing magnitude in the city. When nursing students are assigned to work with youngsters in schools, they very often are accepted as role models and mentors. Taking this responsibility seriously, they encourage high school students to establish career goals and finish their education before starting a family. They teach growth and development and contribute to health and science classes. In addition, they work with students who aspire to health careers and inspire some to continue in these educational efforts.

The students have implemented health promotion curricula, such as the Basic Aid Training (BAT) program developed by the Red Cross for elementary school children. This course presents basic responses to acute situations and can be taught during the term in weekly sessions. Students who have taught these classes have stayed involved with the children in the schools, and some groups have worked with a class during their 4 years in the health centers. During this time they have been able to assess the growth and development of the children and their families, and learn about the developmental tasks of each group age. The nursing students also may work in day camps or summer programs with children, and some have become involved in playground safety, organized clean-up campaigns, or lobbied for improvements in the recreational equipment.

Secondary Prevention

Students make many home visits and learn about the varied structures and roles in families today. Recent immigration patterns have led to extended families living under one roof or in several apartments in one building. Elder housing has created separate environments in which formerly independent residents are "aging in place" and in need of increasing services, as they are living apart from their families. People with AIDS often have extended networks of caregivers or same-sex partners who comprise their family. Students become adept at adapting to the health care needs of the neighborhood residents and are very creative in their strategies to deliver nursing care. Because the students have the time to spend with families, they develop in-depth knowledge of their concerns. Some of these family relationships span courses, and the students continue to learn from and be involved in a family's care throughout their educational years.

One area for community interventions with families occurs in the health status indicator of preventable hospital discharges. These are defined as conditions that could have been treated in primary care settings so that hospitalization might have been avoided. In the city of Boston there are three highly prevalent conditions for which data are available. Asthma is found at the top of this list, with a rate of 424.1 hospital discharges per 100,000 residents. This rate compares poorly with the state figure of 266.7. Since the Healthy People 2000 goal is 160.0, this is clearly an area for family education about limiting the effects of this illness (MDPH, 1994).

Students have been actively involved in community needs assessments about services and education to control asthma. They have been placed in asthma clinics and have contacted patients who did not keep their appointments to determine how best to meet their needs. They have made home assessments of the presence of allergens, and they have developed teaching tools that identify areas for clarification during the clinic visit. In schools, students have conducted classes about the care and use of inhalers and provided medication cards and teaching for children.

The second most prevalent preventable illness is bacterial pneumonia. The rate of hospitalization for this infection in the city of Boston is 288.3, whereas the state the rate is 223.1 (MDPH, 1994). Students have conducted record reviews of seniors receiving adult day care and/or home care to determine if they have had flu vaccines; they have organized clinics to provide immunizations. For homebound elders, the students have made home visits for flu injections, and have held clinics at housing sites for the elderly throughout the city.

A third major category of illness is angina. Students have been very active in the elder services network and have conducted exercise programs, nutrition workshops, and blood pressure screenings to prevent exacerbations of illness from coronary artery disease. The students have taught medication management to seniors and caregivers and focused on proper use and storage of nitroglycerine. They have worked with the visiting nurses assigned to elderly housing units to obtain lists of medication that their patients are receiving, have made home visits to teach elders about their prescriptions, and have assessed their ability to comply with their medication regimes.

Tertiary Prevention

Students have been very involved with shelters for the homeless in the city and have become aware of the complex needs of homeless families. They have worked in clinics in the shelters and helped staff mobile vans that canvass the city to deliver health care and education to people on the street. Through this work they learn about complex health care needs in this population that spans all ages. Clinical assignments also include soup kitchens, meal sites, and overnight shelters. After observing the need, students have conducted clothing and food drives and participated in immunization clinics for the shelter guests. They have worked with outreach workers and coordinators to find homes for these clients. Assessing nutritional status, the risks of environmental exposure, infectious diseases, and skin integrity have all been a part of their clinical learning. In fact, students have learned the importance to health of many of the environmental manipulations that Florence Nightingale taught in Crimea.

TEACHING/LEARNING

According to the Massachusetts Department of Public Health (1994), the leading causes of death in Boston are heart disease (28.7%) and cancer (23.2%). When the students develop teaching projects, they can look at the life-style, behaviors, and risk factors that may be amenable to change in order to prevent these conditions. Using a list of diseases and the related risk factors may provide insights into the many health promotion projects that the students can offer the community. In the process of developing their projects, they learn about the illness and the measures one takes to prevent or ameliorate the symptoms.

In Massachusetts in 1992, one-third of deaths were attributed to heart disease. Students learn about the pathophysiology and treatment of heart disease and also about the risk factors and behavior patterns that may be amenable to change in the community. Smoking cessation programs, stress reduction workshops, nutrition and exercise classes, and increased physical activities for all age groups have been advocated by the students in their health promotion programs. Cholesterol screening and blood pressure clinics have also been conducted, for young and old alike. Referrals are made to the neighborhood health centers for follow-up when needed.

The second leading cause of death in the state is cancer, which accounted for over 25% of the deaths in 1992. The students conduct environmental and occupational assessments for carcinogenic substances in the community. Their physical assessment skills incorporate inspection and palpation for possible tumors. The effects of diet, tobacco, alcohol, and sun exposure are all topics covered in health classes in the schools or for parenting groups.

This strategy may be followed for the other leading causes of death, cerebrovascular disease, pulmonary disease, accidents, and infectious disease. This is one way that nurse educators can incorporate the health promotion and disease prevention aspect of community care into clinical teaching.

COMMUNITY

After repeated clinical experiences within the neighborhood, students identify strongly with the community and its needs. By being assigned to one neighborhood during their clinical nursing education, they have come to know its leaders and have collaborated with many community members. One goal of this program is to help students become more comfortable with these residential areas, electing to return to these communities to work after graduation. In some cases, students have moved into these neighborhoods; others have chosen to affiliate with health centers near their homes.

During their educational experience, students are taught the principles of prevention and are oriented to focus on individuals, family, and community. As students look at individual goals within the expanded framework of the community, they can see that changing individual behavior will have an effect on normative public health practices within the community.

Although the data presented in this chapter reflect the incidence and prevalence of disease for the city of Boston, the students who are working within each neighborhood recognize the local variation in demographic variables and have identified community needs and priorities. Because of their longevity in the neighborhoods across the courses of the curriculum, their understanding of the value of health promotion and disease prevention is deepened. By the time they reach the community course, they are able to apply the science of epidemiology and look at the effects of prevention on the current health status indicators and the associated risk factors that relate to an increased incidence of disease, disability, and other health problems in their community assessments. They are ready to expand their focus and to view their neighborhoods within the broader context of the city and the state.

Some students elect to conduct community assessments in other neighborhoods than the ones in which their health center is located. In doing this, they discover the local nature of particular concerns shared by neighborhood residents and the variations in leadership within the community that are mobilized to address these conditions. By experiencing other neighborhoods, often within the role of the visiting nurse, the students gain another perspective and acknowledge the disparities that exist in our current system of health care delivery. Students often use their knowledge of resources to create linkages across systems and can bridge gaps between health and human services. They bring their knowledge of community resources and an interdisciplinary focus to care planning and case management. In gathering resources within the community, students are able to provide leadership. As they develop their projects, such as health fairs, they work with key members of the community to encourage the participation of formal organizations and grass-roots interest groups that reflect the ethnic, racial, and cultural diversity within the neighborhood. They are able to consider other social, economic, and political groups in the community, including those outside the traditional fields of public health and health care delivery.

Access to health care services is improved when there is more than one gatekeeper into the system. Through their involvement with religious, educational, legal, and recreational services within the neighborhoods, students bring health promotion and disease prevention activities to a broader population, using existing resources. This is seen through the clinical activities in the mental health course, in which psychopathology is taught within the context of family and community life. When mental health concepts are integrated into the problems that exist in our society, many of the destructive behaviors in schools and on the streets can be understood. Students develop preventive interventions in conjunction with teachers, social workers, probation officers, guidance counselors, and pastors. One example of this sort of collaborative effort is the peer leader program in the city. The rising crime rates among youth, gang violence, and drug abuse were areas that were targeted for improvement by the neighborhood health centers through these peer leader programs. The coordinators for the peer leaders are funded by the Suffolk County district attorney from the drug money that is confiscated by the criminal justice system. Peer leaders are adolescents or young adults who are community residents; they receive training in conflict resolution, group process, program development, and leadership skills. The nursing students have joined these groups and added the dimension of health promotion education. The nursing students, because of their own youth and ability to set and achieve goals in their lives, have been valuable assets as peer leaders and role models in their work with troubled youth in the neighborhoods who have the potential for violence and gang activities.

The students have also spent time in residential treatment facilities and shelters for the homeless. Even beginning-level students have made a positive impact on the clients. For example, one group of students in a battered women's shelter identified the low level of self-esteem among the residents. They offered the women a session on hair care and cosmetics. The students brought their knowledge of hygiene and sense of style to the group. The residents' feelings of self-worth and beauty were heightened, and the session turned out to be very therapeutic. The students also took photographs of the women so that they could see themselves as others see them. This activity was the basis of ongoing intervention and therapeutic communication for the residents of the shelter. The mental health counselors were also engaged in these activities and guided the students and residents when feelings were shared.

When students enter the neighborhoods initially, there is a period of adjustment during which they identify the local human, physical, and financial resources for health promotion. The presence of students helps to promote change, as they are able to engage the community in disease prevention efforts and provide an essential base on which outside resources can expand. For example, students can provide the staffing that is needed for mandated screenings in schools. The public health nurses in the school system often cover more than one site and have heavy demands for medication administration, tube feedings, and catheterization. Some are providing daily treatments using nebulizers and chest physical therapy. Students are excited to have the opportunities to learn technical skills and can work in conjunction with the nurse to conduct the blood pressure, height and weight, and vision and hearing tests that must be done. They are also taught to conduct scoliosis screening by the health educator or physical therapist.

There is a reciprocal service component to this type of clinical education because of the extra time that is taken from community providers' schedules to meet the learning needs of the students. As providers work with the students, their participation in this educational process may actually extend their ability to provide health care to their aggregate populations. With prolonged engagement in the settings, the school nurses have obtained videos and educational programs that the students conduct in the classrooms. Working with groups of principals and school boards, the students have developed and participated in health education curricula for the school system in the community. These activities have helped to solidify the relationships between the students and community members. Another mutual benefit is in the sense of ownership and commitment to enhanced health care in the neighborhoods through education of the students.

Neighborhood participation is key to initiating change and then maintaining the momentum. Students' progression through the curriculum and vacation breaks can disrupt this process. As community leaders come to appreciate the benefits achieved by having students, they are creating community jobs for them, enabling them to sustain their work when school is not in session. Some students work in residential shelters for abused women and have taken the course for telephone crisis intervention. They committed a certain number of hours to volunteer for this telephone time; then a position was created for them so that they could maintain continuity with these residents. After graduation one of these students was recruited by a shelter in another neighborhood to supervise such a program.

Besides the creation of jobs to keep the students actively engaged within the community, reciprocal relationships have been created between the university and the neighborhood. Nursing faculty practice in the neighborhood health centers. Providers within the health centers have been recruited and hired as part-time clinical faculty, and community residents who teach the students consistently have been appointed as adjunct faculty of the university. By recognizing in more formal ways the contributions of local people to this community-based curriculum, the sustainability of these efforts can be enhanced. The importance of joint planning and shared participation cannot be overemphasized in the process of bringing about enduring changes in health care delivery patterns that will promote healthful conditions in the ways neighborhood residents live, work, learn, worship, and use leisure time. The notion of the partnership between the residents of the neighborhoods, the staff at the health centers, and the faculty and students at the university is a bond that must be continuously nurtured if these programs are to be sustained and successful.

Another tenet in teaching about prevention is the recognition that there is no such thing as a "quick fix" solution to problems. An ongoing commitment is necessary for disease prevention within the neighborhoods. The model of education described here is not clinical nursing in a different location or a community health course integrated throughout the curriculum. The participation of each member of the partnership is necessary if these programs are to be ongoing. At the same time, prevention programs must evolve and adapt to an ever-changing environment and community-based needs. This means that standardization of student experiences across neighborhoods or across courses is not possible. Therefore, the curriculum threads must be broad-based enough to meet the educational needs of the students and be flexible enough to incorporate the dynamic nature of the community. Community needs are developed from sound epidemiological research and program evaluation findings. Continuous evaluation of students and faculty expertise in health services research provides ongoing study of the effects of this curriculum on the students and residents of the neighborhoods.

TARGETING PUBLIC HEALTH GOALS

As faculty seek ways to improve and refine the education of students in community health, concerns have been expressed about the differences between community-oriented education and education that is truly community-based. When students are community-oriented, they have clinical experiences in the community and seek to understand community systems. This differs from a community-based curriculum, in which students' clinical practice is created in partnership with the residents in the neighborhoods. Each of these levels of practice affects the health of the community because the students are working with the population of the community to meet their identified needs. The goals of the Massachusetts Department of Public Health (1994) outline the broad, target areas for public health of the commonwealth, and the student community clinical experiences can be created to fit within these categories. Student clinical activities are targeted at certain risk behaviors to promote more healthful life-styles within the following objectives.

1. *Slow the progression of HIV.* This objective will be measured by reducing the number of inappropriate hospitalizations by providing a range of community support services to HIV/AIDS clients and implementing disease prevention initiatives to slow or stop the spread of HIV infections among individuals who are practicing high-risk behavior. The nursing students have worked extensively in the school systems to provide health education about sexual development and the hazards of unprotected sexual activity. The prevention of teen pregnancy and parenting education programs for young mothers are other clinical experiences aimed at reducing the number of those at risk. As students educate others about the risks of HIV, they become more aware of their own risk in potential occupational exposure. Students have led informational sessions within the health centers and for community groups about routes of possible transmission. Because of their active involvement, the students stay up to date on litera-

ture and research in this area. The HIV coordinators in the health centers have been instrumental in the students' heightened awareness and understanding of this disease.

2. *Prevent drug and alcohol abuse.* The prevention of drug and alcohol abuse among the young is another area in which the students have been heavily invested. Working with established groups, such as Mothers Against Drunk Driving and Students Against Drunk Driving (MADD and SADD), students have led groups and conducted informational sessions in schools and community health fairs. In one program, the students brought in advertisements for cigarettes and alcohol that were aimed at young people and pointed out the real dangers and health risks to the students. During that same week, a sports journal was distributed to the students in the fourth grade that was full of these advertisements. When the students returned to the school the next week, the children rushed over to tell them about the journal and its sponsors. The nursing students were pleased that the children had remembered their presentation and reacted to these advertisements negatively.

The students have also worked with police and the legal system in educational sessions and participated in group sessions under the auspices of Alcoholics Anonymous. Many of the problems seen within families and the neighborhoods can be traced to alcohol and substance abuse. The students have been involved in prevention, early intervention, and treatment services. With the youth of the community, students may have the strongest impact through their role modeling. Especially for boys whose fathers may be absent and who learn through peer pressure and gang behaviors, the young men who have chosen nursing as a career have been very influential in presenting another worldview, influencing others to set and achieve goals and stimulating thought about other careers. The cycle of drugs and violence becomes a daily maintenance cycle, which often prevents future planning and goals. The exercise of goal setting and building self-esteem through developing ongoing relationships has characterized the work that the students have done with youth groups in drop-in centers and schools.

3. *Improve healthy birth outcomes.* Another state public health goal is to reduce low birth weight and infant mortality and disability. Students have addressed concern is through targeting the

adolescent population for teenage pregnancy prevention and becoming involved in community outreach efforts to women of
other cultures, who often do not come into the health care system
for prenatal care. Another is through the Women, Infants, and
Children (WIC) programs for nutrition education. All students
have clinical experiences with the nutritionists and outreach
workers in this federally funded program. Students become very
knowledgeable about the parameters for eligibility and the process for applying for these benefits and routinely incorporate this
into their care plans.

   4. *Improve the health of children, adolescents, and women.* The
public health objective is aimed at developing comprehensive services addressing the particular health and developmental needs
of these vulnerable groups. WIC experiences, shelters for the
homeless and abused, and early intervention, pregnancy, and
parenting programs are all aimed at the needs of women and
children. Day care centers, youth organizations, summer camps,
and the teen peer leader programs are other sites that have welcomed the students. Schools are very receptive to the nursing
students' ongoing involvement and health promotion events. Because students are involved in these community organizations,
they become adept at recognizing risk behaviors and can intervene before illnesses develop or at earlier stages of family disrup-
tions.

   5. *Prevent disease.* This is another target area for public health.
The goal of improving surveillance and control of communicable
and infectious disease can be seen with the HIV population and
also with flu clinics and tuberculosis (TB) tracking. Several
groups of students have become engaged in record reviews for
TB testing and follow-up and have summarized data for the
health centers on how many clients return to have their tests read
and what follow-up has been provided to increase the numbers
of people who do. The students have also made links between
the health centers and the Department of Public Health for staff
education about the services provided for TB care. Students have
followed residents for compliance with the long-term therapy required to treat active disease. They also have spent clinical time
in the inpatient facilities to provide care for those with a need for
more complex health care or structure to control the transmission
of TB.

6. *Minimize harmful environmental exposures.* The students are also taught about occupational and environmental health. They learn about protection of the public, minimizing exposure to unnecessary microbiological, chemical, and physical hazards in food, drugs, medical devices, pesticides, and consumer products. One very interesting student experience involved research about peak flow meters that the health center wished to purchase. The students undertook the project and contacted local hospitals to find out which brands they used and which were given to patients at discharge. They learned about the features of each brand, the costs, and whether they were designed for a single patient to use or could be sterilized in the health center between patients. They discovered how reliable the measurements were across the various brands. They put all their research together in a presentation to the clinical directors and administrators at the end of the term, with plans for a staff in-service education program and the development of protocols for their care when the peak flow meters were purchased, Patient instruction guidelines and recommendations for a home visit to assess for environmental allergens were also recommended by these students.

These objectives of the Department of Public Health are designed to promote the availability and accessibility of quality health care services in Massachusetts while working to control health care costs. The allocation of scarce resources is always a concern when programs are planned in health care. From their first clinical course, students become aware of the economics of health care; they must include a budget in their planning process and incorporate a cost/ benefit analysis in their evaluations. These evaluations contribute to establishing the benefits of community clinical experiences to the community, especially in the areas of health promotion, which are currently not reimbursable by many third-party insurers.

The students provide a significant degree of help to meet the goals of the state Department of Public Health by improving access to care for vulnerable populations, especially women and children. They have developed outreach and treatment services, using culturally appropriate and neighborhood-based strategies to meet locally identified needs. Students have been able to implement and expand prevention and intervention services beyond the scope of the professional providers in various settings within the community. In so doing they have enhanced access to health care services for hard-to-reach clients, including men and women with disabilities, the homeless, and the underserved. By working within the neighborhoods they have been able to individualize health care services for cultural and linguistic minorities and people of color. These strategies have helped faculty and students in the community-based clinical curriculum to maintain and improve the quality of health care and prevention services by conducting evaluation studies, promoting systematic program monitoring, and developing need indicators to access areas of greatest need.

But probably the greatest benefit of this model of nursing education has been in the holistic perspective of the students. By their active involvement and participation in the lives of residents of the neighborhoods, students gain a true sense of community health. They become increasingly sensitized to the needs of the population they serve. Through this educational experience, students and residents have been able to build and mobilize coalitions to achieve the goals of a healthier community. Leadership is shared between the partners, and institutions collaborate with grass-roots constituencies to achieve mutual goals. Because of this involvement, providers do not develop a sense of discouragement or indifference to the complex care needs of the underserved but instead have a sense of communal sharing of responsibility for meeting those needs. It is an empowering process that will lead to the formation of a new generation of creative clinicians.

SUMMARY

As nursing students progress in their professional development, they may be jointly guided by university faculty, community leaders, and professionals from a variety of disciplines. Students are able to explore areas of interest in more depth and not only develop nursing skills in communication, critical thinking and nursing therapeutics but also become more expert in the care of a certain condition or population. Clinical learning is enriched when activities develop in an evolving progression, based on on-going assessment and expanding skills and lasting beyond the single session but even beyond the single course. Educational outcome objectives are achieved, and students are simultaneously allowed to individualize their programs so that they may contribute their unique abilities to the process of meeting the health care needs of a specific population. Students enjoy the sense of achievement such supported independence provides experience the responsibility and comfort that long-term affiliation offers, and graduate aware that they are able to function within a broader scope of nursing practice than they had previously anticipated.

REFERENCES

Massachusetts Department of Public Health. (1994). *Health status indicators: Community health network areas, Metro Boston region.* Boston: Author.

7

Evaluating the Program's Impact

Peggy S. Matteson
Carole A. Shea
Mary Anne Gauthier
Barbara R. Kelley
Margaret Ann Mahoney

Started in September 1991, the program at Northeastern University has evolved and grown. From the start the changes have had a pervasive effect on the college of nursing and the participating communities. These effects will be examined in this chapter from the point of view of the students, the faculty, and the community. We will describe our expectations for the program and contrast these with the program's real outcomes.

During the process of curriculum change and program development, goals and outcomes were set for the curriculum as a whole and then for each individual course within the curriculum. Clinical instructors, working within specific neighborhoods, developed additional goals for each clinical group, and students were also assisted in setting their own individual goals.

EFFECT OF APPROACH ON NURSING STUDENTS

Anticipated Outcomes

Anticipated outcomes focused on the knowledge, skills, and attitudes that students would attain from participation in a longitudinal clinical experience within a neighborhood as part of their overall plan of clinical experiences.

Knowledge

To provide nursing care within a community setting students must have a knowledge base that is different from the knowledge base developed for hospital care. The knowledge of nursing therapeutics remains the same; however, differences occur in how to access the health care system; how to identify and access the clients; how to provide care when you are a guest within the community environment; how to develop a therapeutic relationship, not only with the client but also with the social support system; and how to provide longitudinal care.

Anticipated knowledge outcomes were an understanding of continuity of care not only as it applies to an individual or family unit but also how it applies to intervention programs developed for a population group; an understanding of health care services offered outside the institution of a health care center; and the knowledge that health care may be provided by extending the traditional boundaries of primary care to include strategies and programs that influence economic, social, and cultural factors of the target population.

Skills

The development of the nursing skills of communication, critical thinking, and therapeutic intervention is a mandate for every nursing education program. With the change in clinical assignments it was anticipated that students would be able to learn technical nursing skills in a variety of sites, some quite different from those used in traditional programs. With creative planning, potential obstacles could be overcome as mechanisms for learning sterile technique, dressing changes, and the administration of medications by various routes were found in community sites.

Simultaneously, other nursing skills would be developed as different interactions were discovered or developed, enabling students to participate in response to community-identified health problems. Through community-based health care projects, undertaken by students in conjunction with faculty and residents, students could learn the basics of communication, health assessment, and critical thinking and develop a skill level that would allow them to function as effective clinicians.

Attitudes

To appreciate the need for an extensive community educational experience, students need to overcome the stereotype of nursing that is projected in the media and develop an appreciation of the broad scope of nursing care (Zungolo, 1994). Many traditional students still enter nursing with the idea that they will graduate, receive a cap and pin, and then help doctors in the emergency department or the operating room. It was anticipated that exposure to the broader scope of nursing practice would broaden students' understanding of the role of a nurse and also lead more graduating students to choose to work in the community.

The changing educational focus also desired to help students view health care as a service delivered in fulfillment of a social contract between the health professionals and community they serve. Through the partnership model of care, students could learn to value the input of the community residents on health care issues, enabling projects to be developed within a context established by the residents.

Effective health care is not delivered by nursing alone but within a multidisciplinary model. It was anticipated that nursing students would develop a strong sense of team if they worked with students from social work, theology, medicine, public health, criminal justice, and other areas.

Actual Outcomes

Developing a mutual educational relationship with a neighborhood has helped provide health services for residents, who reciprocate by participating in the education of nursing students. When the members of a university come into a neighborhood and learn about it and its problems from residents, a constant unveiling of reality occurs. This shared experience fosters creativity, creates an interactive process in the development of the structure of educational experiences, and enhances the students' development in the process of utilization of self. Through this process, students, faculty, neighborhood health care providers, and participating residents achieve what Bellah and associates (Bellah, Madsen, Sullivan, Swidler, & Tipton, 1985) have described as two of the most basic components of a good life: success in one's work and the joy that comes from serving one's community.

The measurement of educational outcomes for students experiencing this process has occurred in two ways. First, qualitative data have been obtained by the students through weekly journals and their evaluation of the clinical experience. Given this mechanism, students can be very frank about how they view their knowledge and skill development and the value of specific learning experiences. Attitudinal change is generally made apparent in a more subtle manner, as students' reflective responses have revealed after exposure to certain experiences. Some students are able to identify these changes within themselves and excitedly report the expansion of their views.

To obtain a measurable evaluation of the actual outcomes of this educational process, a comparative study was designed. Its purpose was to compare the views of two different groups of seniors graduating from the college of nursing. One group (n = 19), admitted to the program before the initiation of change, experienced only traditional clinical placements. The other group (n = 32), admitted as the changes started to occur, experienced not only hospital-based placements but also a longitudinal placement within an urban neighborhood, which continued across clinical courses.

The tools were selected because of the attributes they measured, as well as their established reliability and validity. They had originally been developed at a time when the assumption was that the hospital is the primary location of nursing practice; therefore, some of the focus of the questions and terminology reflect this bias. Responding to a faculty concern that the students with increased community placements would not be as well prepared as traditional students, this was not considered a problem. The hypothesis was that there would be no difference between the two groups of students.

Data were collected using three instruments: the Six-Dimension Scale of Nursing Performance (Schwirian, 1978), the Lawler-Corwin Nursing Role Conception Scale, modified professional subscale (Lawler, 1988a), and the Lawler-Stone Health Professional Attitude Inventory (Lawler, 1988b). These three instruments allow comparison of students' views concerning the nursing role, their professional attitudes, and self-assessment of preparation to provide nursing care.

Knowledge

In the beginning of their educational program some students, who focused on future employment within hospital settings, expressed concern that a program with 50% of the clinical experience outside the hospital would limit their scope of knowledge development and they would not be prepared for a hospital position. They verbalized these concerns less frequently to faculty members as they moved through the program, and by graduation they seldom expressed them.

As students gained a broader view and working knowledge of health care as a system they came to understand how learning about care in the community could enhance the care they provided hospitalized patients. As students became able to provide appropriate collaboration and referrals, the discharge planning they provided to hospitalized patients improved. Students developed an understanding that the knowledge of community resources and routes to access of care made them better prepared as nurses.

The knowledge attained by students is measured in a variety of ways within each course of a curriculum. Students in the two tracks of the comparative study took the same courses and were taught by the same faculty but attended the courses at different times. Evaluation of the academic performance of these two groups of students was provided by the same structure and mechanism within each course. There were no reports from faculty about obvious differences in the end-of-course evaluations of the students of each group.

Comparisons were also made using state board results and employment. Results of the state boards indicate no significant difference in the pass rate of students even though the questions on the exam are more focused on institutional acute care than on health promotion and disease prevention.

Finding a nursing position in the era of nursing cutbacks is always difficult. Breaking into such a job market may be facilitated though professional networking. After their long-term interactions with professionals in the neighborhoods, the community-based students were helped in their search for employment by referrals from the clinicians who had educated them. The community-based students offered a broader variety of skills to potential employers than those students whose clinical experiences were primarily in acute care settings.

Skills

Some students initially expressed concern that with so much clinical time within a community setting they would be unprepared to perform the technical skills required by hospital employers. They were concerned not so much about obtaining a position as a registered nurse after graduation but more urgently about obtaining employment as a nurse's aide while still in their educational program. Lack of skills has not been a problem. In fact, by the end of their sophomore year students have completed the required hours of didactic instruction and technical skill development required to qualify for home health aide certification. What has slowed some students' employment has been a lack of understanding on the part of hospital employers that students may obtain these skills in an environment outside the hospital.

By the completion of the nursing program, students who had participated in the community clinicals placements did not express the concern that replacing the hospital environment with a community environment had handicapped their professional educational achievements. In fact, some found that they were more employable than their classmates who had participated in the traditional program because they offered more diverse skills.

Evaluation of students' technical abilities may actually be enhanced by neighborhood placements as increased opportunities exist for students to practice technical skills. For example, when students participate in a flu clinic for the elderly, they interact individually with their instructor as they provide multiple injections. After students have administered 15 or more injections sequentially during a 3- or 4-hour clinic they have not only learned a skill but also simultaneously developed a sense of confidence in their ability to perform the task independently. Even students who were very anxious at the start of a session became more relaxed and developed a sense of competence with repetition. This is a very different learning experience from the one provided in an inpatient hospital setting in which the student cares for the needs of only one or two patients. The same benefits in skill development were also achieved through other community programs, such as blood pressure, serum glucose, and tuberculosis screenings. In fact, the intradermal injection technique was reintroduced into the curriculum because of the demand for services.

The development of clinical skills within courses for the two groups of students compared in the study were taught and then evaluated during different quarters but by the same group of faculty for each course. No differences in final evaluations of students' abilities were reported by the faculty.

Students' perceptions of the adequacy of their nursing school preparation for nursing practice were compared at the completion of the program by use of the Six-Dimension Scale of Nursing Performance (Schwirian, 1978). Five subscales explored clinical competence in the areas of interpersonal relations/communications, leadership, critical care, teaching/collaboration, and planning /evaluation. Items in the interpersonal relations/communication subscale relate to interpersonal relationships and communication with clients and colleagues in the health care setting. The leadership subscale addresses leadership activities an individual would perform regardless of the job title. Items in the critical care subscale relate to nursing activities associated with the care of very critically ill individuals, including the potential outcome of death. The teaching/collaboration subscale addresses the nurse's roles of teaching clients and families and collaborating with a patient's family and other care providers. The fifth subscale, planning/evaluation, addresses the planning and then evaluation of the outcome of nursing care. Including all five subscales, the instrument contains 42 items in which students rate their own ability on a 4-point rating scale, ranging from not very well (1) to very well (4). Comparative analysis indicated that there were no significant differences in levels of confidence between the two groups of students. An educational experience with decreased time in acute care facilities did not lead students to report less confidence in their ability to provide a full scope of direct nursing care, even for the critical care category.

Attitudes

Attitudinal changes generally, take place gradually making them very difficult to evaluate in process. However, some situations dramatically illustrate a student's change in attitude and motivation. For example, one student showed some reluctance in the clinical groups' learning activities, remained quiet during discussions, and implied that she did not expect to learn much about nursing during the experience. To complete her clinical work she was required to participate with classmates in a teaching-learning project, providing health teaching in an elementary classroom. The topic was substance abuse. During the course of the presentation one of the children shared with the class the fact that his mother was a drug addict and explained in detail how this had affected his and the whole family's lives. He also expressed his appreciation for an aunt who had taken him and his siblings into her home. At the end of the child's very emotional presentation, the nursing student softly replied to the child, "Isn't it wonderful that you have an aunt to take care of you and love you." After this classroom incident the attitude of the nursing student changed dramatically. She became enthusiastic, passionate, and engaged in her clinical activities. During her reflections on the experience she expressed surprise that, even with so many problems to overcome, these children were still bright and motivated. This encounter changed her view of the neighborhood residents and their need for nursing services. With new respect she saw how important her nursing care could be in the lives of children and became an avid participant in community-based nursing education.

One desired attitudinal change of the program was that more graduating nurses would consider employment within community settings. It was hoped that some would enter that arena of care immediately after graduation and that others would view it as an option later in their careers. To determine graduating students' plans for future employment they were asked, "In what type of health care setting do you anticipate that you will be working during the next year?" and "What do you picture yourself doing professionally five years from now?" Of the students who identified an employment site, all of the traditional students (100%) and the majority of the community students (93%) anticipate employment within a hospital setting for the next year. This was a higher percentage of community students than faculty anticipated.

In response to where they expected to be professionally in five years, 21% of the traditional students and 38% of the community students identified working in a community setting. The traditional students' aspirations were tied to becoming nurse practitioners. Many of the community students also desired to become nurse practitioners; however, others stated they simply wanted to be a nurse working within a community.

These responses of students were not as heavily slanted toward community work as faculty had hoped. The reasons may be based on two different phenomena. First, the students who comprised the community group decided to enter nursing before the health care debates of 1993–1994. Their views of nursing care were probably developed in a fairly traditional manner. Therefore, despite exposure to community nursing within this program, many retained the original vision that led them to become nurses. This was validated by statements from some students that the community assignments were just something they had to "get through" to graduate. Several students threatened to sue the university or leave the school in order to receive a more traditional education. Neither of these events occurred, but they demonstrate the degree of unease some students felt with the new clinical focus.

Another explanation of why community students generally chose to seek hospital employment first appears in some of their statements explaining their professional aspirations for the next 5 years. Of those students who desired to eventually work in the community, one-third stated that they had to obtain at least 1 year's experience on a medical-surgical unit before they moved on to another position. This statement is heard repeatedly from many practicing nurses and nurse educators. With hospitals downsizing their nursing staffs, 1 year on the medical-surgical floor can no longer be the gateway for entry into practice. More to the point, with health care moving to the community there is an increasing need for nurses competent in this arena to provide services. Students who complete a curriculum with both hospital experience and a longitudinal component of community care are capable of fulfilling many community positions without a year of hospital-oriented care. Some community agencies are hiring students with the broader clinical experiences straight from school.

Beyond their choices of where to seek employment, other attitudinal differences between the two groups were explored. For comparative purposes, measurement of attitudinal differences was provided by two instruments, the Lawler-Corwin Nursing Role Conception Scale (modified professional subscale) (Lawler, 1988a) and the Lawler-Stone Health Professional Attitude Inventory (Lawler, 1988b).

Lawler-Corwin Nursing Role Conception Scale

The modified professional subscale of the Lawler-Corwin Nursing Role Conception Scale (Lawler, 1988a) addresses traditional professional attributes, independence of practice, and standards of excellence. Each of the 14 items describes a hypothetical situation a nurse might encounter in practice. Respondents are asked to indicate the extent to which they think each situation "should be the ideal" in nursing practice and then the extent to which the described situations "actually do exist" in nursing practice. Each item is answered on a 5-point Likert-type scale ranging from strongly agree (5) to strongly disagree (1). In response to the hypothetical situations the traditional students achieved a slightly higher mean score in both the ideal of nursing practice and observed nursing practice. The community students responded with a broader range of scoring to both the ideal and observed nursing practice. There was no significant difference between the ideal or actual mean scores of the two groups of students. An interesting phenomenon occurred when two of the respondents in the community group attained negative discrepancy scores, which indicated that for them the observed nursing behaviors were more professional than their ideal.

The degree of noncongruence between actual and observed nursing practice is calculated by subtracting each respondent's actual score from his or her ideal score. Mean scores for the two groups may then be obtained and compared. Comparison of the professional role dissonance or discrepancy score of each group indicated no significant difference between the two groups of students.

Lawler-Stone Health Care Professional Attitude Inventory

The Lawler-Stone Health Care Professional Attitude Inventory (Lawler, 1988b) contains a series of statements about today's health care professions and health care delivery systems. It measures attitudes toward six aspects of professionalism: consumer control, concern with credentialing, subordinate purpose (concern with well-being of others and human welfare), critical attitude (questioning and skepticism toward traditions and established practice in health care), impatience with rate of social change, and compassion (dedication to the care of others). This inventory contains 38 items to which participants respond on a 5-point Likert scale, ranging from strongly agree (1) to strongly disagree (5).

Scores for the total inventory showed no significant differences between the two groups. Differences were revealed only when the mean subscale scores were compared. The most significant differences were found in the subscale scores of compassion ($p = .03$) and consumer control ($p = .05$).

Compassion

The subscale compassion measures a health care provider's compassion for the needs of the client and public and dedication to care for others. At a level of significance of .03 the community students scored higher than the traditional students. Item analysis determined that significant differences in responses occurred on three of the seven questions of this subscale. These statements were (1) "Policies based solely on scientific methodology are most appropriate for the resolution of society's health care problems"; (2) "Health care teams tend to become so busy coordinating care that they lose sight of patient needs"; and (3) "Health care is currently available to people at differing income levels on a selective basis."

In response to the first statement, "Policies based solely on scientific methodology are most appropriate for the resolution of society's health care problems," twice as many traditional students as the community students were undecided. When the response categories of agreement and disagreement were collapsed respectively, 71.88% of the students who had spent more time in contact with community providers disagreed with the statement, whereas only 47.37% of the traditional students responded in the same manner. The community-based students were reacting from a broader experiential focus. On the basis of their educational experiences, they may have ascertained that the appropriate response to society's health care problems requires a more human-centered, holistic approach than scientific methodology permits.

Students' responses to the second statement, "Health care teams tend to become so busy coordinating care that they lose sight of patient needs" also demonstrated that the two groups had opposite response patterns. The combined "disagree" and "strongly disagree" responses for the community students (40.63%) almost paralleled the "strongly agree" and "agree" responses of the traditional students (47.37%). The opposite responses may be attributed to the fact that the community students participated in health care teams that performed in a different manner from that of the teams the traditional students were exposed to in hospital settings.

Similarly, the third statement, "Health care is currently available to people at differing income levels on a selective basis," led to responses that were almost exactly reversed. On the basis of their patient contact experiences, which occurred primarily within hospitals, 47.37% of the traditional students agreed or strongly agreed. The patients they care for, by virtue of their hospital admission, had some way in which to access the health care system. Conversely, of the community students who had repeated patient contact in neighborhood sites, as well as in hospitals, almost the same percentage of students (46.67%) disagreed or strongly disagreed with this statement. Perhaps this difference may be explained by the fact that community students provided health care to a variety of clients in a number of sites and participated in providing free care. In a nonexclusionary manner they provided health care in places where neighborhood residents work, gather for social events and worship, attend school, or play.

Consumer Control

The subscale for consumer control measures the variable of a student's commitment to consumer control and collaboration in health care decisions. In an unexpected finding the traditional students scored higher in this subscale ($p = .05$). Because of the clinical work the community students had accomplished in collaboration with community residents, this outcome was surprising. Item analysis explored students' responses. No significant differences were revealed between the groups except in their responses to the following statements: (1) "Health care professionals have actively encouraged consumer participation in current delivery systems" ($p = .002$) and (2) "Education programs for health care professionals are currently designed to prepare professionals who will be able to appropriately respond to the needs of the local community" ($p = .077$).

Community students have had more opportunity than traditional students have had to work with health care professionals providing care in a broad spectrum of sites. With a greater exposure to different types of providers, students have a broader experiential base from which to answer this question. In response to the statement "Health care professionals have actively encouraged consumer participation in current delivery systems," more than twice as many traditional as community students were unsure about the phenomenon and responded with the choice "undecided." Of the traditional students who made a decision, 42.1% disagreed or strongly disagreed with the statement. These students seemed to believe that health care professionals have not encouraged the participation of consumers. The community students who made a decisive choice were almost evenly divided in their responses, with almost as many agreeing (37.5%) with the statement as those expressing some degree of disagreement (40.63%).

The statement "Education programs for health care professionals are currently designed to prepare professionals who will be able to appropriately respond to the needs of the local community" deals with the design of current educational programs. The majority of community students, participants in a nursing education program designed to change nursing education for just this purpose, responded with a majority of agreement and strong agreement (59.38%). Traditional students, who were not participating in the program but were being educated within the same college of nursing by some of the same faculty and were most likely aware of the educational changes, responded with a total agreement of 47.37%. Perhaps close interaction between the two different tracks of student groups influenced their responses, or possibly students of each group were not able to discern whether they should respond based on the basis of the program they were participating in or the other program they knew existed.

EFFECT OF APPROACH ON NURSING FACULTY

From the initial response to the Kellogg request for proposals to the unanimous faculty vote to proceed with the submission of a full application, the faculty of the College of Nursing was invited to participate with other members of CCHERS in the developmental process. Once site selection occurred, faculty continued to be included in various development and implementation activities.

Anticipated Outcomes

It was expected that changing the curriculum of the College of Nursing was a task to be shared among the complete faculty. The administration anticipated that the implementation process would require possible changes in skills, knowledge, and/or attitudes on the part of some faculty members. The desired outcomes for College of Nursing faculty were as follows:

1. The faculty would teach a major portion of the clinical experience for nursing students in the neighborhood health centers and other community-based settings.
2. The faculty would collaborate with community providers in making clinical assignments and developing community-based learning projects.
3. The faculty would work in partnership with community providers and residents to teach the principles, skills, and values of community-based primary care to nursing and other health professions students.
4. The faculty would develop institutional and professional connections between the College of Nursing and the neighborhood health center to build a community-based academic health center for education, research, and service.
5. The faculty would participate in community-based primary care, research, and service.

To achieve these outcomes, faculty members needed a broad knowledge base that crossed disciplines. Knowledge of community, primary care, empowerment, collaboration, culture, conflict resolution, epidemiology, health professions education, and teaching methodologies are just a few examples of the content areas underpinning the new approach to nursing education. Likewise, faculty members needed to draw on principles, science, and research related to health promotion and maintenance, as well as disease processes and acute care interventions.

Similarly, a broad array of skills was necessary. Faculty members would have to be able to structure a clinical learning experience that would take advantage of different activities and projects in different locations. (A student group would no longer practice in a single unit or agency but could be assigned throughout a community.) The nurse educators would have to be able to work as part of a clinical team in designing, delivering, and evaluating the clinical portion of the curriculum. Skills involved in making comprehensive assessments of individuals, families, and communities were required.

The values supporting the new approach are not unique to nursing but require setting different priorities and emphasizing some beliefs more than others. The foremost goal was to provide education to prepare health professions students to deliver culturally appropriate, community-initiated, comprehensive, high-quality primary health care. To accomplish this goal, it was necessary for faculty members to embody the values inherent in cultural diversity, community empowerment, collaboration, health promotion, and disease prevention. Further, they would need to demonstrate the appropriate attitudes through their words and actions by giving priority to educational activities that support students' learning of these values.

Actual Outcomes

The effect of the new approach to nursing education on faculty was more profound than originally thought. It was anticipated that faculty would become more culturally sensitive, more knowledgeable about community systems and services, and more invested in ensuring access to primary health care through their involvement with students, providers, and community residents in neighborhood health centers. Over time this did occur, but the scope and depth of new knowledge, skills, and attitudes that some faculty members needed to successfully implement the community-based primary care curriculum were underestimated.

After identifying knowledge and skill deficits, a plan for "faculty development" was then created to assist in the achievement of desired outcomes. Faculty members were surveyed to determine their learning needs and teaching interests. Based on the survey results and goals of the project, faculty development seminars and workshops were offered to all faculty involved in the project. For example, workshops were designed for academic and community faculty members to teach the development of cultural competence in students and how to take advantage of a "teachable moment" in a busy clinic, resolve conflicts, and build teams and collaborative networks. These workshops were taught by faculty from within and external to the project. For unidentified reasons most of the workshops were not well attended. However, those who did participate indicated that the workshops were informative and useful. Possible reasons for poor attendance may have been resistance to change, inability of individuals to identify themselves as needy, a lack of release time for educational programs, or scheduling conflicts with an individual's teaching assignment.

As the project proceeded, it became evident that the diverse faculty had many additional learning needs. For example, some nurse educators lacked the knowledge, skills, and attitudes necessary for entering into the life and health care of the community, for socializing students to the role of the professional nurse in the absence of caregiving nurse models, and for sharing the teaching role with community residents, other professionals, and nonlicensed workers. Others had some of the fundamental knowledge and skills but were unable to apply them in the new settings. The time and encouragement to adopt new attitudes and values had to be given further consideration.

Considering the sweeping nature of the new curriculum, it was not unreasonable to assume that there would be some unintended consequences or unanticipated difficulties with the new approach to curriculum. However, the amount of anticipated difficulty tended to be obscured by several working assumptions already in effect. The assumptions that were found to be not entirely true were the following:

1. The new curriculum would be a return to the historical roots, philosophy, beliefs, and practice of nursing, which

emphasized holistic, continuous *health* care of individuals, families, and communities. It was envisioned that, at last, nursing faculty would be able to teach and do what they said they valued most.

2. The faculty already possessed the requisite knowledge, skills, and attitudes to teach the new curriculum; they would be able to apply them in the new community-based settings.

3. Although the new approach would fundamentally change the nursing curriculum (e.g., the content and methods), it would affect the nursing faculty only indirectly. Therefore, faculty members would need to focus on the process of implementing the curriculum rather than their own learning needs or other faculty-related outcomes.

4. The benefit to the faculty would be the greater opportunity for integration of their full role of teaching, research, and practice through collaboration with others within a community-based setting.

As the project proceeded, each of assumption was challenged by the forces of reality. For example, some nursing educators found it difficult to give up their focus on content and skills better suited to acute care in tertiary settings. Many had difficulty accepting the underlying premises of a health-oriented curriculum, preferring to teach what they knew best—aspects of specialty practice in a hospital setting. Even the community health and primary care faculty found that application of their expertise required modification when teaching undergraduate students in neighborhood health centers.

Before students can become empowered, faculty must be freed from the constraints of tradition. The college administration must provide support and resources to facilitate the development of creative approaches in generating clinical assignments. As individual faculty members move toward developing alliances within neighborhoods, they need the opportunity to collaborate with others who are pioneering in new clinical arenas. Mutual support and information sharing make the process of development even more dynamic and fruitful.

College faculty role-model expected student behaviors. When

exploring and developing possible neighborhood experiences, faculty members also develop a working relationship with a multidisciplinary team of providers, community workers, and community residents. When students are brought into the arena, they follow the faculty member's lead on how to relate to the community partners. Reinforced within this collaborative model is the theme that everyone has something to teach; everyone has something to learn (Gauthier & Matteson, 1995).

The primary changes in health professions education were designed to benefit students by preparing them for a new system of care that would provide consumers with better access, quality, and efficiency of health care, thus benefiting society as a whole. Benefits for the faculty, who were viewed as the means for achieving this outcome, were more indirect. As a result, less attention was given initially to faculty preparation for new roles. Despite the faculty workshops and seminars, specific outcomes, with attendant objectives, content, method, strategies, and evaluation, were not a priority of the project. In essence the nursing faculty was expected to concentrate on curriculum development collectively and identify and address personal learning needs and professional outcomes individually. Some faculty members succeeded in taking this approach, whereas others struggled to remain apart from the process.

The actual outcomes of the new approach to nursing education for faculty who became actively engaged in the change process were very positive. They embraced curriculum adaptations that focused on health promotion and disease prevention; shifted the venue of clinical teaching to community-based settings; provided a longitudinal experience for students to work with families and the community; reframed undergraduate clinical learning to include comprehensive assessments, health teaching, health counseling, multidisciplinary projects, and seminars; and collaborated with community providers and residents in providing educational experiences for students.

Faculty members, some in their fourth year of collaboration with a neighborhood, are developing a more thorough understanding of their neighborhood's needs and resources. Community members and providers seek them out for assistance with research concerning health problems or program development, implementation, and evaluation. Several have been able to integrate their full faculty role, conducting research and providing service within their clinical community. What started as a project has now become integrated throughout the College of Nursing, enabling an increasing number of faculty members to make progress toward the anticipated outcomes.

In retrospect, advancement toward the project goals might have been realized more easily if the outcomes for faculty had been given a greater priority and more advanced planning had occurred. Faculty members' integration into the educational changes required strategic planning and more resources to attain new knowledge, skills and attitudes in a systematic way in order to carry out this substantive curriculum change.

EFFECT OF APPROACH ON COMMUNITY RESIDENTS

Educators have the ability and obligation to reform nursing education so that it provides students an opportunity to learn about the range of diversity within majority and minority cultures. The development of a partnership with community residents through a longitudinal neighborhood clinical experience helps bridge "the dichotomies that exist between the world we teach about and the world people inhabit in everyday life—the world in which the people we care for live" (Chopoorian, 1990, p. 26). Through the experience, clients become partners in the education of nursing professionals.

Anticipated Outcomes

Even though the curriculum change was occurring within the structure of College of Nursing, it was anticipated that these changes would have an impact on the residents of the neighborhoods and their health.

Knowledge

The improvement of the health of residents within a neighborhood is dependent, first, on the accurate assessment of past attempts and current needs and, second, the provision of health care initiatives to facilitate these self-identified needs. The involvement of individuals, families, and community leaders is essential in determining the problems of the community and how they might be most appropriately addressed. Input from clients and the community must be given value in determining the content and style of the care they receive. Within this collaborative process, appropriate nursing interventions can be developed, not only to provide direct care but also to expand the resident's knowledge about how to improve their health status.

By providing additional staff for health care planning and intervention, the nursing students and their faculty are able to assist in the building of a sustainable system of health and human services based in neighborhood settings. With an expanded knowledge base and assistance in the development of programs, community residents can become capable providers of certain levels of health care.

Skills

Many community members, both residents and providers, possess a variety of skills that nursing students must learn. Tapping into this expertise and structuring the nursing students' interactions so that they may learn from other disciplines enrich the students' overall learning experience. Community providers who interact with students as mentors and teachers are offered adjunct faculty status.

Community providers, already established and respected within the neighborhood, offers a model of the desired attitudes and behaviors required of nursing students and faculty. Learning appropriate behavior right from the beginning facilitates the acceptance of the "outsiders" by the neighborhood and enhances the learning experience.

Bringing the expertise and resources of the university into the neighborhood allows faculty to work with members of the community to formulate research questions and investigate phenomena specific to the community. This partnership could expand the research abilities of clinicians within the neighborhood.

Attitudes

Community clinicians' and residents' skepticism about their value and ability to teach nursing students can be overcome by assisting them to identify their unique knowledge base and structuring mechanisms through which they may impart that knowledge to nursing students and faculty. As comfort and ease with the teaching of nursing students increases, providers can assume increasing responsibility for initiating educational processes with students.

Residents living in the identified communities are empowered to teach students also. Drawing on their lived experience, these individuals offer a unique knowledge base to the students. Students learn from the residents about their lives, concerns, and difficulties with health care. For collaborative purposes, community members and leaders are incorporated and integrated into various aspects of the educational process.

Actual Outcomes

Enlisting the support of community members, whether clinical staff, community workers, or residents, is a slow process that first requires the development of trust. Asking members of an economically depressed urban community to share their knowledge with student nurses is a relatively new concept. Community providers and residents have been "burned" in the past by short-term, self-serving institutional commitments and are rightfully hesitant to believe that the new focus on a joint educational experience is any more than lip service.

Knowledge

Community residents provide an expertise in the neighborhood's history, the cultural diversity among members of the community, the functioning of the community, and/or the prioritized needs of the community. For example, one community had been identified by outside sources as having a high rate of infant mortality. Exploration with community residents determined that they were aware of the severity of this problem, yet they prioritized violence prevention as the problem they wanted to address. They believed that with the decrease of violence some of the blocks to prenatal and pediatric care would be reduced, thereby leading to reduction in the number of neonatal and infant deaths. Once the community representatives and the members of the College of Nursing reached an agreement to work toward the reduction of violence, the community members became receptive to the development of additional health care interventions. Knowledge about how to approach residents and their contacts within the community is valuable for the students. The development of the flu clinics for the elderly is another example of success due to joint planning.

The influx of students into the health care arena of a neighborhood has provided additional service hours and expertise in health care services. Students have increased the amount of health teaching in schools, provided more home visits than paid employees of community agencies can supply, and provided valuable one-to-one care to vulnerable clients when agencies were unable to provide such services.

Skills

A large variety of competent clinicians were found within the neighborhood. With encouragement, they have provided additional mentors for nursing students. Teachers have shared knowledge of how to engage a classroom of children and present material in an age-appropriate manner. Social workers have demonstrated the techniques of a home visit and interviewing. Ministers have taught students how to approach a client and develop a therapeutic caring relationship.

Explaining the educational experiences required and desired by students and then jointly determining how these needs may be met within the community provides validation that the college faculty truly views this as a partnership. When members of the community work in this manner, students develop a realistic notion of the needs and abilities of community residents and learn to view community residents as valued members of the educational team.

Nursing practice and nursing education, although complementary activities, are two distinct cultures. Those who inhabit each of these worlds have different ways of doing, exploring, and learning. Enlisting the support of providers of nursing care within the neighborhood has been essential. Explaining how this educational approach is different from what they themselves might have experienced was critical. Once they understand the concepts of the program, health care providers determine for themselves how best to share the expertise each has developed in providing care within the neighborhood.

Research questions raised by community practitioners and community organizers have led to partnerships with university faculty. Both graduate and undergraduate students have participated in various steps of the research process. Several quality improvement projects have been completed that resulted in changes in the delivery of care. Other collaborative research has been completed in the form of pilot projects that are now being expanded for more extensive exploration through grant funding.

Attitudes

Because of past experiences, both providers and community residents have been understandably slow to change their attitudes. Full acceptance by some is apparent; others are helpful yet guarded. Now that the presence of students has continued over a number of years, the sincerity of this partnership initiative is in many ways less suspect. However, there are still those who wonder out loud if there is a limit to the commitment of the College of Nursing.

Nevertheless, in increasing numbers, members of the community, both providers and residents, have volunteered to become partners in the educational process and have made a commitment to share their concerns and lives with students. Organizers and participants in programs for the elderly, schools, and other community-based services have requested the service of students. The inclusion of nursing students increases the extent of available programs despite limited budgets. Individuals themselves often ask organizers when the students are returning.

Within some of the health centers, acceptance of and collaboration with students has been more sporadic. Not all individual providers have felt a responsibility to interact with students or share their knowledge and expertise. Some view students as an imposition that slows down their workday. Others do not wish a student to observe them when they are interacting with clients. Fortunately, there is a gradual increase in provider acceptance, yet the pace is slow. Sharing time with students was not included in the job description of many of these employees when they were hired, and they do not feel a sense of responsibility.

The presence of students in the neighborhood has increased the number of health care services provided in many measurable ways. What is less measurable is the question of whether their presence has changed the attitudes of residents with regard to health care. Two examples indicate that to some degree this has occurred.

At day care centers, individual students spend a number of weeks as classroom nurse. One student became involved with a 5–year-old boy for a period of time each week. He was very active and responded best during one-to-one interactions. After the student had fulfilled her obligation at the day care center, she began working in the pediatric clinic of the neighborhood health center. Quite by accident this child was one of the clients she was assigned to care for. When he saw her, he yelled to his mother, "That's my nurse!" The nursing student was pleased that he remembered her and then served as his nurse during his well-child examination. At the completion of the exam, the clinic staff remarked at how well the child had behaved for the nursing student. This was a first, as previously the child had been extremely fearful. At no prior visit had the staff been able to attain as much assessment data or provide interventions with such ease. For the first time, a clinic visit was not a traumatic experience for this little boy, because "his nurse" was with him and coordinating his care.

Another example involves the program participants at a senior center. These participants range in age from mid-50s to mid-90s, with the majority between ages 70 and 90. The director of the program has observed that since her clients have been able to spend time interacting with nursing students, they have become less hesitant to seek health care. The nursing students have spent a great deal of time listening to these elders as they learned about their lives, health care problems and concerns, and culture-specific health care interventions. The elderly have had the value of their self-report validated by the students' careful attention and now appear at the health center with more expedience when they have health concerns.

Community residents and health care providers are increasingly valuing the nursing care provided by students. Because of the success within the four initial neighborhoods, additional communities requested that they be considered for inclusion in the program.

SUMMARY

Developing and implementing a community-based curriculum in which the community is a partner in the educational process are challenging yet rewarding experiences. Some goals of this project have occurred with less difficulty than expected; others have been more difficult to achieve. The process has also provided some desirable yet unexpected outcomes. New professional alliances and friendships have been formed across employment sites. A sense of shared accomplishment has developed as successes were celebrated and difficulties approached with fresh vigor.

Students have reached graduation as well prepared for implementing the skills of clinical practice as traditional students are. In addition, they possess a sense of accomplishment when they are able to evaluate for themselves the difference their efforts make in the lives of a specific community and they possess knowledge and attitudes that will enable them to practice more competently within a rapidly changing health care system. This longitudinal stay within one clinical location has provided them with the chance for success in work and the joy that comes from serving an adopted community. As a result some students have moved directly into employment opportunities within community-based programs.

Faculty members have been challenged by these curriculum changes. Some readily accepted the positive challenge and worked to implement the idea of a community-based curriculum. Implementation has been an ongoing process as educational strategies were developed, utilized, and evaluated. Because each neighborhood is a unique entity, different approaches work in different areas. Supporting each other's endeavors and allowing time for joint brainstorming has enabled faculty to be very creative in the development of neighborhood clinical sites. Because of the full support and encouragement offered by the administration, these faculty members have been able to create an educational process that some thought was impossible to achieve. Such involvement leads to a professional satisfaction and the development of many new collaborative relationships for research and practice.

Community clinicians and residents have also benefited from participation in this program. Services have been provided that were previously unavailable. Providers have obtained the assistance of developing professionals to aid in the delivery of care. Some clinicians have added a new dimension to their professional practice as teachers of the providers of the future.

REFERENCES

Bellah, R., Madsen, R., Sullivan, W., Swidler, A., & Tipton, S. (1985). *Habits of the heart: Individualism and commitment in American life.* New York: Harper & Row.

Chopoorian, T. (1990). The two worlds of nursing: The one we teach about, the one that is. In *Curriculum revolution: Redefining the student-teacher relationship* (pp. 21–36). New York: National League for Nursing.

Gauthier, M. A., & Matteson, P. (1995). The role of empowerment in neighborhood-based education. *Journal of Nursing Education, 34* (8).

Lawler, T. (1988a). Measuring socialization to the professional nursing role. In O. L. Strickland & C. Walsh, (Eds), *Measurement of nursing outcomes* (vol. 2, pp. 44–46). New York: Springer.

Lawler, T. (1988b). Measuring socialization to the professional nursing role. In O. L. Strickland & C. Walsh (Eds), *Measurement of nursing outcomes* (vol 2, pp. 46–49). New York: Springer.

Schwirian, P. (1978). Evaluating the performance of nurses: A multidimensional approach. *Nursing Research, 27*(6), 347–351.

Zungolo, E. (1994). Interdisciplinary education in primary care: The challenge. *Nursing and Health Care, 15*(6), 288–292.

Epilogue

Eileen Zungolo

Since 1989 the College of Nursing at Northeastern University has responded to many internal and external changes. This book has described the process used to develop a model of undergraduate nursing education that is in and of the community, and specific illustrations of how to develop such learning experiences in neighborhoods.

UNDERGRADUATE CURRICULUM

The development and implementation of an undergraduate curriculum that would support the mission of the university, meet the educational needs of the students, and serve the health care needs of Boston residents has been a major task. The curriculum evolved from a progressive program of study geared to the rich clinical learning resources of Boston's acute care community, including an innovative health promotion and disease prevention framework encompassing primary care needs in a community-based approach. The implementation of this new curriculum has facilitated students learning in the changing health care environment and has fostered greater collaboration with neighborhood providers and residents. The College of Nursing is committed to continuing to strengthen this collaborative educational process.

COMMUNITY PARTNERSHIPS

While identifying and defining these learning experiences for nursing students, we have also made a substantial investment in the growth of the coalition between the educational institution and our neighbors through development of the Center for Community Health, Education, Research, and Service (CCHERS). The development of this partnership has required participants to have a strong commitment to primary care and a belief in the right of all residents to accessible health care. Needed as well was the vision that professional nurses could make a difference in these outreach efforts and that basic nursing education should prepare nurses to practice primary care that is community-based. With these values we forged new relationships, established procedures and guidelines, and engaged multiple agencies and neighborhood residents in the process. In short, we have built a comprehensive liaison between the academy and the community. The College of Nursing is committed to sustaining these efforts and exploring additional joint ventures.

New initiatives continue to emerge as previous goals are realized. As our students, faculty and their relationships with the community function with increasing ease, other projects have become viable. Our next steps will take us beyond the immediate needs of academic programs. Although the bulk of our attention over the past 4 years has been on curriculum development, we are now moving to improve community services, conduct research, and extend our education mission.

EXPANDED COMMUNITY OUTREACH

One of the initial and continuing concerns of our neighbors has been their desire to build a relationship with the academic community in order to broaden the opportunity base for their children's educational advancement. Concurrently, the College of Nursing has lamented our inability to meet the learning needs of some minority students. Efforts to enhance opportunity for some students usually involve remediation efforts to address the inadequacies of prior educational experiences. As nurse educators we have long regretted our inability to influence education at the high school level and even lower. Our community partnership has provided the opportunity to embark on just such an effort.

Recently the Boston School Committee announced a request for proposals (RFP) challenging members of higher education, businesses, and others, to develop creative approaches to education. In collaboration with our partners in CCHERS, the Healthy Transitions/Healthy Futures program at New England Medical Center, and two Boston high schools, we have initiated the development of a Health Careers Academy as a pilot high school. This will inaugurate a program planned to foster interest in careers in the health professions among the children in our inner-city partner neighborhoods. Beginning with four cohorts—a 9th-grade and an 11th-grade classes at two inner-city high schools—this comprehensive program will include academic course work, career guidance and development, family support, internships, experiential learning and employment in health care settings, and participation in university activities. The participants' learning experiences will include work with nursing and medical students in the CCHERS community outreach network in neighborhoods in which the children live.

INTEGRATION OF THE GRADUATE PROGRAM

At the other end of the educational spectrum and of equal importance within the College of Nursing is the desire to integrate graduate program offerings into a community-based approach. Through the partnership we will be expanding the involvement of graduate students in the neighborhood health centers. Graduate students from a variety of specialties will have the opportunity to become engaged in research and service activities. In the past some nurse practitioner students have worked with individual preceptors at partner neighborhood health centers. However, the development of longitudinal experiences will enable students to develop depth in their relationships within the community and expand their learning activities.

Other specialty areas of graduate study will also strengthen their community base. The deinstitutionalization of health care mandates that nurses in other specialties broaden the focus of their concentration to include care in the community. For example, the most common approach to studying nursing administration is to examine nursing departments in a hospital or other acute care facility This specialization now needs to prepare nurses for leadership roles in the management of ambulatory and community outreach services as well.

EXPANSION OF RESEARCH AND SERVICE

The name of the Center for Community Health, Education, Research, and Service suggests that participants will give equal attention to all elements. The curriculum work was the first step in developing, within primary care settings, academic health centers that can function as hubs for research, service, and learning in the same manner that the hospital has in the past. We are now extending and expanding our attention to research and service projects that can be provided by faculty and students. Some research projects, identified by community residents, providers, nursing faculty, or students, have already begun to emerge from within the neighborhood health centers and are being investigated by nursing faculty in collaboration with neighborhood health center staff.

Even with the positive contributions of the undergraduate students, there remain serious health and social problems threatening the integrity of the neighborhoods. As managed care rapidly becomes the major financial backing for health care in Massachusetts, potentially dangerously short hospital stays, with poor follow-up, are threats to health in the neighborhoods. This is necessary to determine the continuing services needed by those who have experienced episodes of acute or chronic illness. The development or enhancement of home health services is one area to be investigated.

Having participated in the establishment of CCHERS, redesigned an undergraduate curriculum, and created a role in the health care services and health professions education agenda of the city and region, we are now eagerly moving to more fully occupy the role and implement the part.

APPENDICES

APPENDIX A
From the Old to the New Curriculum

Carole A. Shea

In 1991 the faculty of Northeastern University (NU) College of Nursing embarked on a journey to develop and implement a new curriculum. The outcome would support the mission of the university, tap the strengths of the faculty, meet the educational preparation needs of students, and serve the health care needs of the Boston community. All while honoring the specifications of a Kellogg grant awarded to create change in the way health professions students are educated.

The curriculum at that time incorporated Roy's Nursing Model, but was heavily weighted toward the "physiologic mode" and disease-oriented medical diagnosis and treatment. Three introductory nursing courses in the first year of study provided basic content about nursing as a profession, the nursing process, and human nutrition. Two fundamentals of nursing courses and a course in pathophysiology followed in the second year. The third year in this 5-year program included a medical-surgical and a psychiatric nursing course. Another medical-surgical course and a maternal–child course were provided in the fourth year. The fifth year included community health, nursing research, contemporary issues, and leadership courses. (See Table A.1 The Original BSN Program for the full curriculum.)

The Center for Health, Education, Research, and Service (CCHERS) consortium, comprised of Northeastern University College of Nursing, Boston University School of Medicine, the Department of Health and Hospitals, and four neighborhood health centers (NHCs), was funded by the Kellogg Foundation to develop academic health centers in which nursing, medical, and other health professions students would participate to learn community-based primary care as an essential part of their practice. It was envisioned that a significant part of the clinical experi-

TABLE A.1. Original BSN Program

	Fall Quarter	Winter Quarter	Spring Quarter	Summer Quarter
Year 1	Human Biology Application of algebra English 1 Introduction to Nursing	General Chemistry 1 Anatomy & Physiology 1 English 2 Nursing Process (L)	General Chemistry 2 Anatomy & Physiology 2 Sociology Nutrition	off
Year 2	**Basic Needs 1 (L & H)** Microbiology Anatomy & Physiology 3 Psychology 1	Co-op #1	**Basic Needs 2 (H)** Pathophysiological concepts Psychology 2 Computer elective	Co-op #2
Year 3	Co-op #3	**Nursing Common Problems (H)** Human Development 1 Pharmocodynamics Peoples and Culture	**Psychiatric Nursing (H)** Human Development 2 Intermediate writing	Co-op #4
Year 4	Co-op #5	**Medical/Surgical Nursing (H)** History elective Humanity elective	**Maternal/Child Nursing (H)** Humanity elective General elective	Co-op #6
Year 5	Co-op #7	**Community Health Nursing (C)** General elective General elective	Intro. to Nursing Research Contemporary Issues in Nursing Leadership & Management Optional elective	

Bold type = clinical nursing courses.
Clinical placement : (L) = nursing lab on campus; (H) = hospital setting; (C) = community setting Co-op = cooperative education placements: most often in hospital settings.

ence of the health professions students (i.e., the request for proposals required at least 25%) would take place in the NHCs that were located in underserved urban areas of Boston and served minority communities. This represented a radical departure for the NU nursing program where the clinical placements were almost exclusively in the tertiary care teaching hospitals of Boston and the Visiting Nurses Associations in the surrounding suburban communities.

The CCHERS group decided to jump start the grant by implementing the proposed plan for community clinical placements in the fall of 1991. To accommodate such a rapid response, the faculty of the college of nursing decided it was necessary that the current courses remain in place with content added to introduce concepts of community, primary care, and culture earlier in the curriculum. However, clinical assignments were changed in the first two clinical courses, placing students in the NHCs during the second year, with additional clinical time in the NHCs as a part or all of their nursing courses in the third, fourth, and fifth years. (See Table A.2 for clinical changes.)

It became obvious to the nursing faculty that consistency in presentation of content would have to be built into the curriculum, particularly the didactic portion of the nursing courses. The clinical experiences in the community settings could not stand alone. Therefore, lectures, textbooks, evaluation tools, skills laboratory sessions—all needed to be developed in support of the learning that was taking place in the community, as well as the hospital.

For the next 3 years the faculty worked on developing an educationally sound curriculum which was futuristic, while at the same time operating a "transitional" program of increased clinical community education. They constructed new courses and negotiated with the other university departments for courses that would be offered in the new curriculum. With community-based primary care outcomes in mind, a curriculum was designed with health as the primary organizing concept. Other changes included balancing community-based and hospital-based clinical experiences, with the community-based ones preceding the hospital-based, to set the orientation toward health. The number of required biology and chemistry courses was decreased in favor of behavioral science courses. The schedule of courses was arranged so that students did not have to take two laboratory sciences (i.e., anatomy & physiology and chemistry) in the same quarter. And there was more flexibility in the way courses could be taken, with fewer prerequisites. In 1994 the faculty came to consensus on the shape and content of the new BSN curriculum. (Table A.3 presents the community-based curriculum plan followed by the new course descriptions.)

Alternatives for implementation were considered. The decision was

TABLE A.2. Original BSN Program with Transitional Clinical Changes

	Fall Quarter	Winter Quarter	Spring Quarter	Summer Quarter
Year 1	Human Biology Application of algebra English 1 Introduction to Nursing	General Chemistry 1 Anatomy & Physiology 1 English 2 Nursing Process (L)	General Chemistry 2 Anatomy & Physiology 2 Sociology Nutrition	off
Year 2	**Basic Needs 1** (L & C) Microbiology Anatomy & Physiology 3 Psychology 1	Co-op #1	**Basic Needs 2** (C & H) Pathophysiological concepts Psychology 2 Computer elective	Co-op #2
Year 3	Co-op #3	**Nursing Common Problems** (C & H) Human Development 1 Pharmocodynamics Peoples and Culture	**Psychiatric Nursing** (C & H) Human Development 2 Intermediate writing	Co-op #4
Year 4	Co-op #5	**Medical/Surgical Nursing** (H) History elective Humanity elective	**Maternal/Child Nursing** (H) Humanity elective General elective	Co-op #6
Year 5	Co-op #7	**Community Health Nursing** (C) General elective General elective	Intro. to Nursing Research Contemporary Issues in Nursing Leadership & Management Optional elective	

Bold type = clinical nursing courses.
Clinical placement : (L) = nursing lab on campus; (H) = hospital setting; (C) = community setting Co-op = cooperative education placements: most often in hospital settings.

TABLE A.3. New Community Based Curriculum

	Fall Quarter	Winter Quarter	Spring Quarter	Summer Quarter
Year 1	Anatomy & Physiology 1 English 1 Application of Algebra Intro. to Professional Nursing Intro. to Career Management	Anatomy & Physiology 2 English 2 Psychology 1 **Nursing Process & Skills** (L)	Anatomy & Physiology 3 Nutrition Social Psychology **Nursing Health Assessment** (L)	off
Year 2	**Healthy Childbearing and Childrearing** (C) Microbiology Sociology	Co-op #1	**Healthy Adulthood and Aging** (C) Pathophysiological Concepts Chemistry	Co-op #2
Year 3	Co-op #3	**Health restoration in Children** (H) Influences on Health /Disease Pharmacology 1	**Health Restoration in Adults** (H) Pharmacology 2 Intermediate writing	Co-op #4
Year 4	Co-op #5	**Promoting Mental Health Restoration** (C & H) Moral problems in medicine Intro. Statistical Analysis	**Promoting Healthy Communities** (C) Medical Economics Intro. to Nursing Research	Co-op #6
Year 5	Co-op #7	**Managing & Leading in Nursing** (C or H) Humanities elective Computer elective History elective	**Comprehensive Nursing Practicum** (C or H) Elective Elective Elective	

Bold type = clinical nursing courses.
Clinical placement : (L) = nursing lab on campus; (H) = hospital setting; (C) = community setting Co-op = cooperative education placements: most often in hospital settings.

TABLE A.4. Comparison of Course Requirements

Original Program	Community-Based Curriculum
Arts and Sciences	*Arts and Sciences*
Anatomy & Physiology 1, 2 & 3	Anatomy & Physiology 1, 2 & 3
Applications of Algebra	Applications of Algebra
English 1 & 2	Chemistry
General Chemistry 1 & 2	English 1 & 2
Human Biology	Microbiology
Human Development 1 & 2	Psychology
Microbiology	Social Psychology
Psychology 1 & 2	Sociology
People & Cultures	Statistics
Sociology	
Core Courses (taught in other colleges)	*Core Courses (taught in other colleges)*
Intermediate writing	Intermediate writing
Pharmacodynamics	Introduction to Career Management
	Medical economics
	Moral problems in medicine
	Pharmacology 1 & 2
Nursing Courses	*Nursing Courses*
Introduction to Professional Nursing	Introduction to Professional Nursing
Theoretical Basis for Nursing Practice	Nursing Process and Skills
Human Nutrition	Nursing Health Assessment
Basic Human Needs 1	Human Nutrition
	Healthy Childbearing and Childrearing
Basic Human Needs 2	Healthy Adulthood and Aging
Pathophysiological Concepts	Pathophysiological Concepts
Nursing Common Problems	Influences on Health and Disease
Psychiatric Nursing	Health Restoration in Children
Maternal Child Nursing	Health Restoration in Adults
Medical-Surgical Nursing	Restoration of Mental Health
Community Health Nursing	Introduction to Nursing Research
Introduction to Nursing Research	Healthy Communities
Contemporary Issues in Nursing	Managing & Leading in Nursing
Leadership and Management	Comprehensive Nursing Practicum
Nursing Electives	*Nursing Electives*
Independent Study	Independent Study
International Health Care Practices	International Health Care Practices
International Health Care Delivery Systems	International Health Care Delivery Systems
International Health Policy Issues	International Health Policy Issues

(continued)

TABLE A.4. *Continued*

Original Program	Community-Based Curriculum
Nurse Entrepreneur	Nurse Entrepreneur
Senior Clinical Practicum	Wellness
Wellness	Women's Health Choices &
Women's Health Choices &	Decisions
Decisions	
Electives	
Electives	
Computer elective	Computer elective
History elective	History elective
Humanity electives-2	Humanities elective
General electives-3	General electives-3

made that the new curriculum be instituted for all students to the extent possible, as quickly as possible in the 1995–1996 academic year. A decision was made to continue to offer two courses from the old curriculum, but only in the 1995–1996 year. The third-year course NUR 1300 Common Health Problems and the fourth-year course 1400 Maternal–Child Nursing were retained to provide content and continuity for those students in the middle of the curriculum. All other courses started with the academic year of 1995–1996. Even so, implemented evaluation and possible revision remain an ongoing process.

APPENDIX B
Course Descriptions of New Curriculum

Course Descriptions

NUR 1102 Introduction to Human Nutrition   **4 QH**
Explores the fundamental role of nutrition in promoting health. Studies the physiological functions of nutrients, their food sources, and recommended intakes for different groups. Uses principles from the humanities and sciences in developing nutrition concepts. Introduces the use of diet assessment tools to assist individuals in meeting nutrient and energy needs. Encourages students to examine their own food choices and how those choices translate into meeting recommended nutrient and energy needs. Discusses the origins of food habits and the relevance of nutrition counseling and education in nursing practice.

NUR 1106 Introduction to Professional Nursing   **2 QH**
Focuses on socializing students to the discipline of nursing with an introduction to theory-based practice and the philosophy of caring. Explores the dimensions of the professional role within the context of the student's developing self-awareness of personal and professional goals.

NUR 1107 Nursing Process and Skills   **3 QH**
Emphasizes the centrality of critical thinking to clinical reasoning. Introduces the nursing process as a problem-solving tool and its application in assessing strategies of communication, gathering data, interpreting evidence, analyzing viewpoints, and forming judgments. Provides scientific principles as the framework for using basic nursing skills in the

practice of selected nursing interventions. Includes practicing skills in a clinical laboratory. *Prereq. or concurrent NUR 1106*

NUR 1108 Nursing Health Assessment 3 QH
Emphasizes dimensions of collecting data relevant to health status. Provides an opportunity for learning to use tools and skills of health assessment. Discusses ethnic, cultural, spiritual, social, psychological, development, gender, and physical aspects of health assessment. Explores formulating nursing diagnosis and examining the relationship of the nursing care plan to overall resources of the client. Includes practicing skills in a clinical laboratory. *Prereq. or concurrent NUR 1107*

NUR 1202 Pathophysiological Concepts for Clinical Nursing 4 QH
Reviews human physiology related to oxygenation, nutrition, elimination, protective mechanisms, neurological functions, endocrine functions, and skin integrity. Explores how the human body uses its adaptive powers to maintain equilibrium and how alterations affect normal processes. Examines disease processes and implications for nursing practice. *Prereq. BIO 1154 or equivalent*

NUR 1206 Promoting Healthy Childbearing and Child Rearing 8 QH
Emphasizes the promotion of health from conception to adolescence. Describes potential and actual health risk factors and explores risk-reduction strategies within the context of the individual, family, and community. Uses the nursing process to provide the framework for students to assess and intervene therapeutically in promoting healthy childbearing and child rearing. Examines the concepts of human development of individual, family, and community within the context of the role of the professional nurse in promoting healthy childbearing and child rearing. Includes clinical learning experiences in a variety of settings. *Prereq. NUR 1108*

NUR 1208 Promoting Healthy Adulthood and Aging 8 QH
Emphasizes the promotion of health in adults and includes common health problems of adults at critical life stages from the young adult to the frail elderly years. Analyzes potential and actual health risk factors and the discovery of risk reduction strategies by applying the nursing process to care of adults living within families and communities. Enables students to use health education and teaching methods in assessing and intervening therapeutically to meet the primary health care needs of adults. Assesses the role of the nurse in partnership with the family and community in disease prevention. Includes clinical learning experiences in a variety of settings. *Prereq. NUR 1206*

NUR 1282 Wellness   **4 QH**
Focuses on experiential exploration of the concept of wellness. Examines behaviors and lifestyle choices that lead to a high level of physical, emotional, and spiritual well-being. Includes issues of assessment of health risk, behavior change, lifestyle analysis, the life cycle, and stress management through self analysis. *Open to any undergraduate student.*

NUR 1304 Independent Study Elective   **4 QH**
Allows students to pursue a topic more intensely or with a special focus. Enables the student to contract with a faculty member whose background, interests, and time allow direction of in-depth study. Requires that student and faculty member jointly develop course objectives.

NUR 1306 Promoting Health Restoration in Children   **10 QH**
Focuses on the therapeutic nursing interventions used to restore health to children who are experiencing acute and/or complex health problems. Analyzes complex health issues within the context of the individual, family, and community. Examines altered family patterns of coping within a developmental framework and describes support to meet the unique health needs of the family and child. Addresses the therapeutic role in partnership with the family and resources available within a collaborative and interdisciplinary environment. Discusses ethical and legal dimensions of caring for children and their families. Includes clinical learning experiences in a variety of settings. *Prereq. NUR 1208*

NUR 1307 Influences on Health and Disease   **4 QH**
Enables the student to understand the values that underlie health-seeking behavior and providing care. Uses values clarification to appreciate individual rights and responsibilities versus the common good. Examines cultural differences in light of individual and group behavior, as well as life-span issues, family, and group responsibilities. Builds a caring ethic and a sense of professional responsibility on the basis of self awareness and self-examination.

NUR 1308 Promoting Health Restoration of Adults   **10 QH**
Focuses on the therapeutic nursing interventions used to restore health to adults who are experiencing acute and/or complex health problems. Analyzes deviations from health with attention to the implications for the individual, as well as the family, in coping with health problems. Analyzes the client's health care needs and the resources to meet them, in collaboration with the client and health providers. Discusses ethical and legal dimensions of nursing care of adults. Emphasizes discharge planning and teaching. Includes clinical learning experiences in a variety of settings. *Prereq. NUR 1206, 1208*

NUR 1404 Nurse Entrepreneur   **4 QH**
Focuses on the role of the nurse as an entrepreneur. Within the general
functions of nursing, uses situations involving patient family teaching
that provide the framework for introducing students to the essentials of
undertaking this function as a business venture. Includes the formation
of a nurse entrepreneur's venture action plan to do patient and family
teaching. *Open to middler students in nursing.*

NUR 1408 Promoting Mental Health Restoration   **7 QH**
Focuses on developing, implementing, and evaluating psychotherapeu-
tic interventions for clients with complex mental health problems. Analyzes alterations in psychobiological and psychosocial functioning and
coping. Formulates a plan of care within the context of the client as individual, family, group, and community. Emphasizes the therapeutic use
of self as students develop communication and other helping skills in
interpersonal relationships with clients. Provides the opportunity to apply theories, principles, and research findings in providing mental
health care for clients in various settings. Fosters collaboration with the
client and interdisciplinary team. Discusses the political, legal and ethical issues related to the delivery of mental health services and the creative role of the nurse. Includes clinical learning experiences in a variety
of settings. *Prereq. NUR 1308*

NUR 1406 Promoting Healthy Communities   **7 QH**
Focuses on developing, implementing, and evaluating therapeutic interventions for the community as the client. Uses the nursing process
within the community context informed by epidemiological trends, so-
ciocultural characteristics, political and legislative influences, organizational programs, environmental factors, and consumer inputs. Emphasizes the role of the public health nurse in multiple arenas of practice.
Examines epidemiological principles and public health policies in relation to identified health problems and conditions in a specific community. Enables students to conduct a comprehensive assessment, in partnership with the community, to develop a program to meet an identified
community health need. Includes clinical learning experiences in a variety of settings. *Prereq. NUR 1308*

NUR 1502 Introduction to Research in Nursing   **4 QH**
Builds on students' prior exposure to select studies applied to nursing.
Discusses and critiques qualitative and quantitative research and the
value of each to the practice of nursing and to the health care field. Examines the importance of research in nursing to both practitioner and
consumer. *Prereq. or concurrent SOC 1320 or equivalent*

NUR 1507 Comprehensive Nursing Practicum   6 QH
Helps students to synthesize nursing knowledge, skills, and experience
and facilitate their transition to professional nursing practice and case
management of clients with complex health problems. Enables students
to demonstrate leadership and collaborative skills in working with other
members of the health care team. Examines professional, role and career issues in a weekly seminar. Includes clinical learning experiences in
a variety of settings. *Prereq. Senior Standing*

NUR 1508 Managing and Leading in Nursing   6 QH
Focuses on the knowledge and skills related to the delivery of health
services within a nursing management context. Presents theories, concepts, and models, such as managed care, organization and management, authority, delegation, resource allocation, budgeting, leadership
and empowerment, change, motivation, environmental safety, quality
improvement, collective bargaining, and conflict resolution, to give the
student an understanding of the knowledge base for the management
role of the baccalaureate nurse. Provides the opportunity to apply principles and practice skills in planning and delegating nursing care using
different organizational models and approaches. Discusses developing
creative roles for managing and leading in nursing. Includes clinical
learning experiences in a variety of settings. *Prereq. Senior Standing*

NUR 1600 International Health Care Practices   4 QH
Introduces the student to the ways in which people in developing nations take care of their health. Considers the cultural context of health
care practices, viewed within a framework of what people believe about
themselves and the world around them; the relationship of individual
and cultural belief systems; the role religious and spiritual beliefs play
in protection, care, and curing; ideas about food and its relationship to
health; the concepts of health education in a belief system; and the ethical issues of health care and resource allocation. *Open to any undergraduate student.*

NUR 1601 International Health Care Delivery Systems   4 QH
Provides students with an opportunity to learn about health care delivery systems in other countries. Introduces the student to a framework
from which to study any health care delivery system. Includes an overview of health care delivery from a variety of perspectives. Investigates
the divergence between two third world and developed nations' health
care delivery systems. Provides an opportunity to study a selected country's health care delivery system in depth. *Open to any undergraduate student.*

NUR 1602 International Health Policy Issues   **4 QH**
Presents a critical approach to selected issues in contemporary international health policy. Includes the socioeconomic context in which such policy arises, the endogenous and exogenous factors that shape it, and strategies that govern its implementation. Examines policies related to a selected issue, such as food and agriculture, in some depth as a model for the conceptual approach to understanding health policy issues. *Open to any undergraduate student.*

NUR 1606 Women's Health Choices and Decisions   **4 QH**
Explores personal health and safety concerns specific to women from menarche to mid-life. Helps to empower students to take charge of their health by examining personal experiences and developing their knowledge base and self-awareness. Investigates self-promotion of health; how to be a knowledgeable consumer; when and how to choose a provider; and care options for fertility regulation, infertility, pregnancy, childbirth, and other conditions specific to women. *Open to any undergraduate student.*

APPENDIX C

Interview with Key Informant

Objective: Student will gain experience and knowledge by interviewing someone involved in the care of the community.

Definition of a key informant: A person who
- knows the community and the health care services provided
- will talk to someone from outside the neighborhood

Procedure to follow:
- Select a person who you think will help you begin to understand the complexities of the agency and the community it serves.
- Explain that you are beginning your clinical rotation in the neighborhood and want to ask some questions. Provide the interview guide if the person wants to think about the questions before you meet.
- If your candidate agrees, make an appointment that is convenient.
- During the interview follow the guide, but feel free to ask other questions.
- Remember that this person is giving up time and energy to help you. Be grateful.
- Write up your findings for your journal and be prepared to share this person's responses with your clinical group.

Adapted from Logan, B., & Dawkins, C. (1986). *Family centered nursing in the community*. Redwood City, CA: Addison-Wesley.

Areas to cover:

- Historical development of site.
    Why was it established?
    How long has it existed?
    Is the need for its services increasing or decreasing?
- Philosophy of organization: care?
- What goals does the organization have?
- Population served: elderly? families? singles? children?
- Criteria for admittance.
- How many clients are served daily? weekly? monthly?
- Hours of operation.
- Health services provided.
- Health services needed.
- Health services met through referrals.
- Source of funding for agency.
- What community outreach services are available?
- What educational events are available to help?
- Are there rehabilitation programs available?
- Are there groups for people with mutual concerns?
- Are there counselors or therapists to help people with specific problems?
- Is emergency care available?
- What health care professionals are available: nurses? psychiatrists? social workers? physicians? psychologists? dentists? podiatrists? other?

What does the key informant see as the health problems of the people who use this agency?

How has the agency responded to meet these needs?

What does the key informant see as the solution?

What does the key informant think are potential health care problems for residents?

APPENDIX D
Cultural Assessment Guide

Conducting a cultural assessment allows you to understand your client and provide culturally relevant nursing care. The following interview guide will provide structure to your data collection by identifying six areas of information. However, adapt the order of your questions and the words you use to the particular client and the setting you are working in. Relax, have a pleasant conversation, and allow your clients to teach you about themselves.

Cultural Affiliation
I am interested in learning more about your cultural background and understanding your health care needs. What is your ethic culture? How long have you and your family been residents in this country?

Health Care Beliefs and Practices
In your culture how do people show others that they care?
  What does care mean to you?
How do you know if someone else is healthy?
  How to you know when you are healthy?
  What do you and others do to stay healthy?
What types of food do you eat?
  How is it cooked?
  When are your meals scheduled?
  Who eats together?
  What have you eaten in the past day?

Adapted from Rosenbaum, J. (1991). A cultural assessment guide. *Canadian Nurse, 87*(4), 32–33.

How do you celebrate special life events (i.e., birth, maturity, marriage, aging, death)?
Who cares for the people going through these processes?

Illness Beliefs and Customs
What is it that causes a person to become ill?
When someone is ill, what does he or she do to get better?
Whom does he or she go to for help? When?
How does a person decide on the need to see a nurse or doctor? Go to a hospital?

Interpersonal Relations
Please think about a small gathering of people of your culture.
Could you describe how they are communicating with each other?
   Are they all talking at once or in turn?
   Are voices loud or soft?
   Are there periods of silence?
   How close do they get to each other? Do they touch?
   What do they do with their hands as they talk?
   Are conversations about things or activities? Are they about feelings?
   What topics are generally not talked about with strangers? Care providers?
How do men and women meet members outside the family they grew up in?
   How do they find someone to marry? Who is acceptable?
   Are their any special ceremonies or problems regarding sexuality?
How do you define a family?
   Are there specific duties for men? For women? For children?
Who cares for the children? Who disciplines them? How is that done?

Spiritual Practices
What are the duties of men and women in your religion and place of worship?
What religious beliefs and practices are a part of your everyday life?
When someone dies, what customs does your religion follow?
   What do you believe happens to that person after death?
   What is the most appropriate way for people to express their feelings to the family of the dead person?
Is anything different when a child dies rather than an adult?

Worldview and Other Social Structures
What part do you play in the world around you? Why is it important that you are here?

What is the most important aspect of your life?

What languages can you understand? Speak? Read?

   Which one did you speak in your home when you were growing up?

What types of jobs have you held? Other members of your family?

   How have finances influenced your life?

Describe the educational experiences you have had. Other family members?

   What educational plans do you have for your children?

There is a lot of electrical equipment used in this country.

   How does it compare to where you lived before?

   How has it influenced your life here?

What have you found to be most disturbing about living here?

What have you found most helpful about living here?

APPENDIX E
Environmental Survey

This survey provides you with an opportunity to learn more about the neighborhood in which you will now be working. Gather subjective data through your personal observations about the residents and the environment in which they live. Use all five senses as you walk and/or drive around the community.

Sight
What did you see when you arrived?
Are there natural or artificial boundaries surrounding the agency? What are the boundaries?
What surrounds the agency? What else is observable from this vantage point?
What is the style of housing? Is everything in good repair?
What transportation is available?
Are there stores: What type: A pharmacy?
Are there schools nearby? Churches?
What recreational facilities are available?
Who do you see on the streets? Children? Adolescents? Older adults? How are they dressed?
Are there any particular ethnic groups present?
Are there any animals around?
Is there any evidence of political activity?

Adapted from Logan, B., & Dawkins, C. (1986). *Family centered nursing in the community*. Boston: Addison-Wesley.

Hearing

What can you hear as you stand outside the agency? Inside the agency?
Does the area seem quiet outside? Inside?
Do you hear children playing?
Are there any loud noises? Music? Machinery? Airplanes?

Taste

Are there any places to eat near the agency? What kinds of foods are available?
Are there any stores for buying food or snacks? What kinds of foods are available?
Did you eat anything? If it was different from your normal diet, describe how it tasted.

Smell

How does the area smell? What does it remind you of? Are the odors pleasant?
How does the inside of the agency smell? Are the odors pleasant?
Describe what you smelled both outside and in.

Touch

Do people on the street look at you? Do the residents seem friendly? Do you feel comfortable?
How do the merchants interact with you?
Are people willing to say hello? Do they ignore you? Describe how you felt.
Inside the agency, do employees seem friendly? Do people say hello? Describe how you felt.

APPENDIX F

Project Proposal Form

Name: Site:

Topic:

Date(s):   Client(s):

Nursing Diagnosis:
(attach supporting S & O data)

Goals:
    Short-term:

    Long-term:

Interventions:

Cost in time: Money:
Evaluation:
   What process will you use?

Evaluation results:

Based on these results, what would you do differently next time? (If necessary use back of page for answer.)

APPENDIX G

Student Clinical Activity Contract

I, _____, will meet with

_____ of _____

on (dates) _____ from (time) _____

at (location) _____ phone _____

in order to _____

_____

_____

_____   _____
Student   Community contact person
home #   work #
work #   home #

_____
date

****

After commitment is satisfactorily fulfilled, please sign, date, and return
to the NU faculty.
Commitment fulfilled on (date) _____
Comments:

_____   _____
Student   Community contact person

APPENDIX H
Outlines of Clinical Activities for Beginning Students

The following are samples of activities developed by university faculty and students, and community providers and residents. They were designed to meet the needs of students during their first year of clinical activity and to start eh professional development of communication skills, critical thinking, and nursing therapeutics. To implement these activities, students are assisted in the assessment, implementation, and evaluation of nursing interventions for individuals, families, groups, and a community.

Site: Client's home
Theme of clinical assignment: Nutritional assessments of homebound.
Design of experience:
 Contact time: 2 hours for 8 weeks
 Nursing students: 2
Objectives:
 For clients
  Review satisfaction with home-delivered meals.
  Identify other health needs.
 For nursing students
  Employ interviewing techniques
  Identify the realities of living within the neighborhood.
  Identify the realities of being home bound.
  Provide referrals for identified problems.
Required supplies/ equipment/ abilities:
 Ability of nursing students:
  Demonstrate understanding that they are guests in the client's home.

Able to conduct an interview while also dealing with distractions and interruptions.

Developmental process:
- Identify an agency that provides home visiting services, such as meal provision, to neighborhood residents.
- Investigate the program and its ability to provide education and supervision.
- Offer the assistance of nursing students.
- Students receive the data collection tool from the home meals agency and learn their interview protocol.

Implementation:
- Students accompany agency employee to view the interview process and be introduced to clientele they will follow.
- Each clinical day the students, working in pairs, meet with supervisor from agency, conduct 3–4 home visits, and then report findings back to supervisor.

  In reference to the meal plan, two examples of what students learned:

  Some recipients did not like the food because it was different from their cultural norm.

  One elderly woman was giving her food to her retarded middle-age son and feeding herself tea and toast.

  Examples of additional findings made possible by home visits:

  A man who required the use of a wheel chair lived on the third floor with no access other than stairs. To go out he threw the chair down the stairs and then eased himself down after it. To return home he crawled up and dragged the chair behind him.

  An elderly resident was being abused by a younger relative and having her monthly check taken in exchange for a bottle of whiskey.
- Students participate in making appropriate referrals.
- Students reassess situation during return visits.

Evaluation:
- Client states the degree of satisfaction with the food.
- Client reports other health care concerns.

- Students improve interviewing skills, deduction of actual or potential problems, and ability to involve other providers.
- Students identify general and specific healthcare needs of neighborhood residents.

- Agency is satisfied with students' written evaluations.

Variation on experience:
- Focus of agency's home visits may be varied.

Hints for success:
- A focused interview involving the completion of a form provides the structure needed for a beginning level students to be successful.

Site: Clinic of neighborhood health center
Theme of clinical assignment: Improving communication skills
Design of experience:
    Contact time: 4 hours for 4 or more weeks
    Nursing students: 2–3 per team
Objectives:
    For clients:
        Continuity of care as provided and facilitated by student and team
    For nursing students
        Employ interviewing techniques
        Utilize assessment skills
        Collaborate within a multidisciplinary team
Required supplies/ equipment/ abilities:
    Equipment: lab coat, personal stethoscope, black pen
    Abilities of nursing students: perform an intake history, assess vital signs, prepare for further evaluation as required, and conduct necessary teaching.
Developmental process:
- Explore possible roles for beginning nurses within the flow of the clinic.
- Explain to other members of the team the students capabilities and their educational objectives.
- Have students oriented to the clinic and the role they will assume.

Implementation:
- Students shadow the provider to learn the role.
- Students assume the role in steps
    Examples of sequencing of students' activities as abilities developed:
        Obtain and review chart then call patient into examination room.
        Learn patient's reason for visit, collect history and perform appropriate assessment.
        Prepare client as needed for continuation of care by nurse practitioner, physician's assistant or physician. Students learn a great deal about the patient's view of their condition and how it affects their life, their expectations of the health care system, their cultural beliefs, the effect of family and commu-

nity on their beliefs, etc., while they wait with the client for
the next provider.

Remain with client through remainder of visit in order to learn
the process and assess how clients needs are meet as they
move through the system.

Students learn about inefficiencies in the system, which serves
two purposes: they understand why clients may become un-
happy with the care they receive and then may collaborate
with the staff to improve services.

Assist in procedures as possible

Two examples are holding children during injections and assisting during gynecological examinations.

Provide teaching and printed teaching material as appropriate
for client's needs.

Assist in referrals to other providers both within and external to
the agency.

Evaluation:

- Client discusses reasons for visit to clinic with student.
- Client responds to student's assessment.

- Student arrives for clinical prepared to demonstrate the skills of interviewing and taking vital signs.
- Student applies concepts and principles of history taking of diverse
clients and evaluates the relevancy of the data.
- Student integrates learning and skills into a plan to assist a client.
- Student appraises interaction and judges the effectiveness of their
interventions.

Variation on experience:

- As student becomes more familiar with the clinic and skills increase he/she is able to assume increasing independence and responsibility.

Examples: obtaining cardiac monitor printouts

participating in telephone triage

conducting nurse clinic visits

Hints for success:

- Share with the staff the educational expectations for the clinical assignment of this level student.
- Match each student to one provider for a clinic session.
- Encourage students to share his/her goals and objectives for each
clinical session with the provider he/she is paired with for the
session.
- Prepare the students for busy times in which providers may forget
to include students in their activities.

- Encourage students to learn the art of staying close to providers without being underfoot.

Site: Day Camp
Theme: Safety in the Park
Design:
   Contact time: 3 hours for 4 weeks
   Nursing students: 4–5 students
Objectives:
   For campers:
      State techniques to improve personal safety
      Apply information to prevent personal injury
   For nursing students
      Apply assessment skills in determining safety hazards
      Develop educational interventions that meet the needs of various age levels
Required supplies/ equipment/ abilities:
   Supplies: paper, pencils, crayons, and other supplies to create mechanisms to reinforce teaching
   Equipment: none
   Abilities of nursing student: beginning health education skills
Developmental process:
   Locate a day camp and offer the services of nursing students for health teaching for a specific number of hours and days.
   Students participate in the camp for a day so they may become familiar with the organizational structure of the program and its participants, as well as assess the developmental levels and possible health needs of the campers.
   Students develop goals and objectives to address assessed risks
   A student (or pair of students) assume leadership responsibility for a specific weekly topic.
Implementation:
   The entire group (of 4 or 5) will participate each week to provide continuity of interaction with the campers
   Plan a topic for each week. For example:
      1. preventing falls
      2. preventing blows to the head
      3. rolling safely (bicycles, roller blades, etc.)
      4. preventing stranger abduction
   The student leader(s) for the week will ensure that the necessary arrangements and supplies are available for the specific intervention
   Campers will be organized into small groups

Nursing students as a group will interact with the campers supporting the student leader(s) in the organized activities

At the end of the camp session the students will conduct a critique of
the week's interactions and prepare with the guidance of the
leader for the following week.

Evaluation:

- Campers are able to answer questions, explain or demonstrate
safety subject matter in an age-appropriate manner.
- Campers related their safety concerns to nursing students.

- Students interact with children in an age-appropriate manner.
- Students conduct a variety of teaching interventions so as to engage the various age levels.
- Students appraise the intervention and judge the effectiveness of
their interventions as they plan for the next encounter.

Possible variations on experience:

Develop program for children on an elementary school playground.

Develop sessions for the counselors on the same topics and provide
first-aid information so they may respond to accidents if they occur.

Hints for success:

Keep the ratio of camper to nursing student at 3 or 4 to 1 by having
multiple groups of campers.

Divide campers by developmental or age levels so level of instruction
can change as the age of the group changes.

Provide a variety of examples and interactive demonstrations.

Encourage the nursing students to work as a team with those scattered among the campers during the presentation, working to
keep them involved with the activity.

All nursing students should assume responsibility for positive verbal
reinforcement of the campers' safety behaviors.

Site: Day Care Center

Theme of clinical assignment: Clean hands

Design of experience:

Contact time: 3 hours per week for 4 weeks

Nursing student: 1 per class

Objectives:

For children

State reasons for washing hands

Demonstrate how to wash effectively

For nursing students

Apply assessment skills to determine health risks of children

Develop and implement age-appropriate intervention
Required supplies/ equipment/ abilities:
Supplies: finger paints or chocolate pudding
Equipment: water table or sinks, hand soap
Abilities of nursing students:
Able to assess and teach children in an age-appropriate manner
Developmental process:
- Locate a day care site and offer services of nursing students for assessment and intervention for a specific number of hours and days.
- Have student participate in at least one session of day care to become familiar with the organizational structure of the classroom and routines of teacher/student interactions.

Implementation:
- Students assess the developmental level and possible health needs of the children.
  Ex. Children did not wash hands after toileting or play, and before eating.
- Students validate assessed need with classroom teacher.
- Students develop intervention with overall goal and objectives.
- Students utilize assistance of classroom teacher in determining appropriateness of teaching techniques and integration of selected theme into other activities of class.
- Students present age-appropriate program.
  Hands of children "dirtied" with finger paints or chocolate pudding used as finger paints. After paint time, children in groups of two or three come to water table to wash hands. Shown process of effective handwashing. Colored "dirt" allows children to monitor their own effectiveness.

Evaluation:
- Children attempt to clean hands in effective manner after painting activity.
- Children wash hands after toileting and before eating.

- Students demonstrate assessment skills.
- Students create and implement an appropriate intervention to instruct the children.
- Students evaluate intervention and plan for follow-up instruction.

Variation on experience:
- Other teaching interventions may focus on basic disease prevention activities such as:
  Use of tissues and covering of nose and mouth for coughing.
  Bathroom behaviors to control spray of urine and proper wiping techniques.

- Assessment of children's lunches may determine need for nutrition education.
- Assessment of play activities may determine safety issues must be addressed.
- As a member of the classroom's teaching team the student may also serve as a health care resource to teacher and provide basic first aid treatment to children.

Hints for success:

- If nursing student is integrated into the classroom before presenting an intervention the:

    Children will respond more readily to the teaching activity.

    Student will know how teacher maintains discipline and be able to evoke same methods.

    Student will be able to evaluate intervention and reinforce this teaching over several weeks.

    Student will have the opportunity for evaluation of other needs and provide interventions as appropriate.

Site: Elementary school
Theme: Learning to relax
Design of experience:

    Contact time: a minimum of 20 hours over 5 weeks.

    Nursing students: 1 student assigned to a specific elementary classroom.

Objectives:

    For children:

        participate in a conscious relaxation activity

        identify how this activity might be used at home.

    For nursing students:

        assess the health of the children, both as individuals and as a group

        develop a teaching/ learning project to meet the needs of the class

Required supplies/ equipment/ abilities:

    Supplies: determined by the activity selected

    Tools: assessment tool to determine children's health information needs (i.e., Van Antwerp, C., & Spaniolo, A. M. (1991). Checking out children's lifestyles, *MCN, 16,* 144–147).

    Abilities of nursing student—comfortable interacting with children and beginning health educator skills

Developmental process:

- Locate an elementary school and offer the services of nursing students for health teaching in specific classes for a specific number of hours and days.

- Have students participate in the class as a teacher's assistant in order to become familiar with the organizational structure of the class, as well as assess the developmental levels and health needs of the students.
- Utilize an assessment process which will reveal health care concerns of the children

Implementation:

- Assess the children's lifestyle to learn their health-related concerns. Assessment indicated that among other things children said they were tired. They explained that they had difficulty falling asleep at night.
- Provide intervention that addresses an identified need(s). Students were led in a discussion of strategies that assist sleep, including conscious relaxation. The students and the teacher then laid on the floor and participated in a conscious relaxation exercise led by the nursing student.

Evaluation:

- Children participate and reach a level of relaxation.
- Children report during their next session if they have repeated the technique at home and are falling asleep more quickly.

- Students use an appropriate tool to assess the needs of the children.
- Students develop an intervention to meet a concern identified by the children.
- Students share the intervention with the children.
- Students evaluate the effectiveness of the intervention in the classroom.
- Students evaluate overall effectiveness of intervention and plan next intervention.

Possible variations in experience:

- Using an assessment tool to determine children's needs can lead to a data base from which a series of health teaching interventions may be developed.
- Other concerns of these children were: oral hygiene, nutrition, exercise, use of drugs, safety precautions, and sense of wellbeing.

Hints for success:

- The children will respond to the nursing student's intervention more readily if they have had at least one session in which the nursing student has participated with the children in the regular classroom activities before conducting assessment and subsequent sessions to provide heath teaching. Multiple visits, just as a student teacher would do, demonstrates that the children are valued as collaborators, not just "guinea pigs" for students' educational endeavors.

- If the nursing student shares the results of the questionnaire with the class the children learn that they have shared concerns and will help the nursing student prioritize their needs.

Site: Homeless—A Food Kitchen
Theme of clinical assignment: Learning from the homeless
Design of experience:
   Contact time: 3 hours per week for 9 weeks. Some facilities require a minimum of a 3-month commitment.
   Nursing students: 2–4 per site. The potential level of experiences provided by the site determines the skill level needed by the student.
Objectives:
   For clients:
      Have opportunity for one-to-one conversation.
      Receive assistance with attaining food.
   For students:
      Summarize the situation of homelessness as identified by those experiencing it.
      Provide assessment of health related needs and appropriate interventions.
Required supplies/ equipment/ abilities:
   Abilities of nursing students: able to use sensitivity in approaching and interviewing individuals who are generally very withdrawn. Once initial contact is made the client must remain in control of the encounter.
Developmental process:
- Locate a facility which provides services to the homeless.
- Offer the assistance of nursing students. Student activities depend on services provided, which may range from a church basement with an evening meal to an overnight facility, with or without nursing clinics. Vans that roam the streets to provide health services and free clinics are also valuable learning experiences.
- Students work as a member of the team providing health care based assessments and interventions.
Implementation:
- Students receive orientation to facility and establish their responsibilities.
- Students participate in the planned activities while evaluating on

an individual level how to develop a sense of confidence and mutual interaction with clients.

Examples of students' activities:

Prepare and serve meals

Conduct informal conversations with clients in order to gain their trust for further interventions.

Provide basic first aid, foot baths or more extensive services if clinic facilities available.

Work with food cupboard and/or clothing cupboard to obtain and provide goods as needed.

- Students participate in weekly seminars to discuss experiences.
- Students follow one or more clients as their case assignment on a weekly basis.

Evaluation:

- Client receives a nourishing meal.
- Clients have an opportunity to interact with students on an individual basis.

- Students improve interviewing skills, deduction of actual or potential problems, and an ability to provided health care as a member of a team.
- Student is able to articulate the complexity of factors that lead to homelessness and demonstrates the ability to apply nursing interventions.

Variation on experience:

- Different locales have addressed the needs of the homeless in different ways. Students may also accompany a team on a traveling health care van or move through the streets taking note of where the homeless live.
- The experience may be varied by the type of site selected, or within larger programs, by the placement of the student within the site.
- As students progress in abilities their responsibilities may also increase.

Hints for success:

- Prepare students for the probable indifference and even possible hostility clients may express when a student sits down near them to talk. Help them not to take it as a personal insult but to see it as a learned response to prior events. Developing relationships with these clients takes a great deal of time.
- Provide frequent opportunities for students to talk about their feelings. They may become shaken as they come to know the clients and realize that they are not very different from them-

selves. Some will be highly educated, some will have jobs, some may be individuals they have known previously before this hardship occurred.

Site: Senior Center
Theme: Monitoring Health Status—Blood pressure
Design of experience:
Contact time: 2 hours for 5 weeks
Nursing students: 1 student/ 4 seniors
Objectives:
For senior citizens:
Repeat value of lower blood pressure
Obtain blood pressure screening and learn individual reading
Recall helpful exercise and diet strategies
For nursing students:
Apply skills of interviewing and taking blood pressure reading
Assess client's individual needs and provide teaching to assist with adherence to medication protocols, diet and exercise
Required supplies/ equipment/ abilities:
Supplies: client-focused educational literature
Tools: stethoscope and sphygmomanometer
Abilities of nursing students: take an accurate blood pressure reading
Provide spontaneous teaching
Developmental process:
• Locate a gathering place for senior citizens and offer to provide health screening, such as blood pressure checks.
• Have each student meet individually with several senior citizens and conduct culturally sensitive health assessments with specific attention to clients' attitudes toward health care providers, diet, exercise, hypertension, and medication. This enables the students to learn from the clients and to have the clients become comfortable with the nursing students.
• Determine if the clients, individually or collectively, have other needs that may be addressed by this group of students.
• Students develop intervention(s) that address the clients' needs and beliefs concerning diet, exercise, and possible hypertension.
Implementation:
• Nursing students use one to two sessions to gather assessment data from clients and the remaining sessions to develop and provide interventions.
• Depending on the needs and abilities of the clients and structure of

the program, multiple interventions may be provided at one session (i.e., a blood pressure clinic with nutrition and exercise information stations) or multiple sessions with a different theme each week.

- Clients with medically controlled hypertension will review drug regimen.
- Clients with hypertension will be referred for further evaluation.

Evaluation:

- Clients are able to recall value of maintaining their blood pressure within normal limits.
- Clients are able to recall personal blood pressure reading.
- Clients state possible improvements to their current diet and exercise regimen.
- Clients with a medically controlled hypertensive condition recall reasons to continue appropriate care.

- Students apply appropriate techniques to conduct a culturally appropriate interview.
- Students evaluate data and provide appropriate teaching interventions.
- Students use instruments appropriately to perform evaluation.
- Students refer clients with possible hypertension to follow-up care.
- Students evaluate overall effectiveness of session.

Value to students:

- Students can learn a great deal about clients and their needs through the preparatory interactions. Rather than coming in as visitors and doing prescribed presentations, the students will develop an affinity for the true needs of the clients by spending time with them.

Variation on experience:

- The health topics to be developed and the types of presentation format to be used are only limited by the imagination and abilities of the students and the concerns and abilities of the seniors.

Hints for success:

- Preliminary interactions in prior sessions are important to the development of the students' knowledge base concerning their clients.
- Development and planning of an intervention should be done in collaboration with interested senior residents.

APPENDIX I

Outlines of Clinical Activities for Advanced Students

The following are samples of activities developed by university faculty and students, and community providers and residents. They were designed in response to an identified health care need, while also providing educational challenges for students as they progress through course activities beyond the basic level. To implement these activities students are expected to be capable of working with increasing independence in the assessment, implementation, and evaluation of nursing interventions for individuals, families, groups, and a community.

Site: Client's home
Theme of clinical assignment: Assisting grandparents with parenting of grandchildren
Design of experience:
    Contact time: 2 hours for 10 weeks
    Nursing students: 2
Objectives:
    For clients:
        Identify community services available to help them and the children
        Identify potential and actual health care problems
    For nursing students:
        Begin the development of a longitudinal, therapeutic relationship with this family
        Employ interviewing techniques
        Assess potential and actual health care problems of family members
        Design and implement appropriate interventions
        Provide referrals as appropriate

Required supplies/ equipment/ abilities:
   Abilities: skills in home visiting, interviewing, and initiative to seek
      out appropriate resources in response to identified needs.
Developmental process
   • Student pair meets with a family identified by community worker
      as being welcoming of and in need of nursing skills.
   • Explore expectations of grandparent for interactions with students.
   • Establish a schedule for type and time of contact.
   • Maintain contact as agreed.
Implementation
   • Each clinical day the students meet with program supervisor to
      plan home visit.
   • Conduct home visit, then review findings and interventions with
      supervisor.
   • Plan a focus for each visit while also allowing time for spontaneous
      interactions.
   • Possible focal points for assessment with examples of students'
      findings:
      Assess the health status and needs of the grandparent
         Stress related to concerns about finances and the physical re-
            quirements of caring for children when own health is failing.
         Conflicted emotions of having to take court action against own
            child for the sake of the grandchild(ren).
         Sacrifice own needs health care needs, time with friends or
            hobbies, food, etc., in order to provide for the children.
      Assess the heath status and needs of the child(ren)
         Many suffer the long term effects of drug exposure during the
            gestational period, neglect, and/or abuse.
         Grieving loss of parent(s).
      Assess the home environment and family needs.
         Retirement income must now be stretched to cover needs of
            growing children.
         Home may no longer be suitable in size or meet the safety
            needs of young children.
   • Develop and collaborate with the grandparent in the provision of
      interventions, including referrals when needed.
      Examples of interventions are:
         Assistance in filing for supplemental income.
         Securing subsidized day care for children.
         Access to health care provided on a sliding fee scale.
         Information concerning free health care program such as immu-
            nizations and screening for children; flu clinics, mammo-
            grams, and gynecological examinations for grandparents.

Access to food banks and federally subsidized school lunch programs.

Obtain from public utilities free supplies and equipment to improve safety in the home.

- Reevaluate previously identified conditions during return visits

Evaluation:

- Students display interviewing skills, describe actual or potential problems, and formulate and implement a plan of care.

- Grandparents express satisfaction with students interventions.

Variation on experience:

- Length of time of interaction with family may be extended beyond initial course up to length of nursing education.
- Selected families may be of any configuration.

Hints for success:

- Development of mutual goals between students and family members is crucial.
- Value family as instructors of their unique view of family and community.

Site: Clinic of neighborhood health center

Theme of clinical assignment: Developing assessment and intervention skills

Design of experience:

Contact time: 4 hours for 5 to 10 weeks

Nursing students: 2–3 students per team

Objectives:

For clients

Continuity of care as provided and facilitated by student and team.

For nursing students.

Collaborate within a multidisciplinary team of care providers

Develop physical assessment skills needed for health screening

Develop educational interventions that meet the needs of the various ages of clients

Required supplies/ equipment/ abilities:

Supplies: informational brochures

Equipment: oto/ophthalmoscope(s), stethoscope(s), Snellen chart, measuring tape, other equipment as needed for clients with specific conditions, such as fetal monitoring devices, glucometers, cardiac monitors, etc.

Abilities of nursing student: beginning physical assessment skills and comfort handling instruments

Developmental process:
- Identify the team(s) providing care
- Negotiate a beginning role for the student(s) within each team. If each student remains with a client throughout the health care encounter more than one student may be accommodated on each team. Observing and participating in the structure the client is moved through makes the students aware of the roles of the various players on the team, what the experience is like for the client, and allows the students to provide continuity for the client.
- Develop a plan for each student to assume greater responsibility in the provision of care concomitant with developing abilities.

Implementation:
- Each student assumes a beginning level role within the team providing care
- As a student's abilities increase so will responsibility for direct care
- Students may identify an area of interest (i.e. a health condition such as HIV+ status or pregnancy, client age such as pediatrics or gerontology, or a case load of clients with conditions to be followed during subsequent clinical day(s), and apply their newly developed skills in the care of these clients.

Evaluation:
- Students meet the clinical objectives of the course.
- Student appraises clinical interactions and judges the effectiveness of their interventions.

- Team members are satisfied with the skill development and collaboration of the student.
- Some clients express satisfaction with the care provided by the student.

Possible variations on experience:
- Clinics may be schedules for a general population or be client specific such as adult, pediatric, adolescent, gynecology; or condition specific such as AIDS, prenatal, hypertension, or emergent care. Each provides a student with a slightly different learning experience while also addressing the development of general nursing skills.

Hints for success:
- Share with the clinical team the educational expectations for the clinical assignment of this level of student.
- Match each student to a team for a series of clinical sessions.
- Encourage each student to share their goals and objectives for this clinical assignment.

- Assist the student to prepare for the assigned experience based on the focus of the clinical assignment.

Site: Day Camp
Theme: How Your Body Works!
Location: Church basement
Design:
Contact time: 3 hours for 6 weeks
Nursing students: 4–5 students
Objectives:
For campers
Recall how specific body parts function
Describe the use of assessment tools
Participate in screening examinations
Identify the role of the professional nurse
For nursing students
Apply the physical assessment skills needed for health screening
Develop educational interventions that meet the needs of various age levels
Required supplies/ equipment/ abilities:
Supplies: paper and crayons for campers to draw their impressions
Equipment: oto/ophthalmoscope(s), stethoscope(s), Snellen chart, tuning fork(s), sensory stimulants for taste and smell, pictures +/ or models for selected body parts.
Abilities of nursing student—beginning physical assessment skills
Developmental process:
- Locate a day camp and offer the services of nursing students for health teaching and screening for a specific number of hours and days.
- Students participate in the camp structure for a day so they may become familiar with the organizational structure of the program and its participants, as well as assess the developmental levels and possible health needs of the campers.
- Students develop overall goal and objectives.
- Have each nursing student assume leadership responsibility for a specific weekly topic.
Implementation:
The entire group (of 4 or 5) will participate each week to provide continuity of interaction with the campers.
Plan a topic for each week For example:
1. heart and lungs

2. eyes and nose
3. bones, muscles and nerves
4. ears
5. "Rap" session

The student leader for the week will ensure that the necessary arrangements and supplies are available for the specific intervention.

Campers will be brought into the room grouped by age and in small groups.

Nursing students will interact with the campers as individuals or pairs at various teaching stations.

At the end of the session the students will conduct a critique of the week's interactions and organize under the guidance of the leader for the following week.

Evaluation:
- Campers participate in interactive dialogue related to their health concerns
- Campers state the purpose of each screening examination

- Students prepare a program of teaching which utilizes a variety of experiences
- Students implement health teaching interventions
- Students answer questions, explain or demonstrate subject matter in a manner that is appropriate to the age of the campers
- Students perform health screening examinations
- Students evaluate findings and refer children as necessary
- Students evaluate teaching techniques and plan appropriately for subsequent sessions

Possible variations on experience:
- Develop program within an elementary classroom
- Develop individual sessions on a specific topic (i.e.—the lungs with interactive stations covering such things as: anatomy of the lungs, lung sounds, smoking cessation, identification and danger of toxic fumes, function of the cough, etc.)

Hints for success:
- Keep the ratio of camper to nursing student at 2:1 by having multiple groups of campers
- Divide campers by developmental or age levels so level of instruction can change as the age of the group changes
- Provide a variety of activities so that students have hands-on and interactive experiences
- Leave a question box with paper and pencils out and available to

campers all week. This provides for answering individual questions and concerns within the small group sessions
- After determining the variety of teaching tools (i.e., charts, models) available, plan each week to have a variety of touching, interactive and thought stations

Site: Day Care Center
Theme of clinical assignment: Illness—identification and response
Design of experience:
    Contact time: 3 hours per week for 4 weeks
    Nursing students: 4 in center
Objectives:
    For parents and teacher
        Describe signs and symptoms of common illness conditions seen at center
    For nursing students
        Apply research skills to locate information on identified conditions
        Develop a teaching tool that is understandable by non-health care personnel
Required supplies/ equipment/ abilities:
    Supplies: paper
    Equipment: access to word processing and duplicating equipment
    Abilities of nursing students: able to locate and compose information in appropriate manner
Developmental process:
- Interview director and teachers at day care center to learn most commonly occurring conditions and their information needs.
- Interview representative parents to learn their information needs.

Implementation:
- Review current consumer focused publications available on this topic.
- Research signs and symptoms of identified conditions. (Teachers and parents identified the following conditions: head lice, scabies, ringworm, impetigo, chicken pox, rubella, conjunctivitis, Coxsackie virus, strep throat, diarrhea, Hepatitis A, and influenza).
- Develop a clear presentation format, create and print tool.
- Review document with health center staff for clarity, comprehensiveness, and suitability.
- Provide an educational program to parents of children and present document to them.

Evaluation:
- Students create an accurate and clearly presented informational document.
- Teachers state the document meets their needs to identify conditions in children.
- Parents state document meets their needs to identify conditions in children and inform them of appropriate treatment regime.

Variation on experience:
- Assessment may indicate a need for further educational documents to be developed such as first aid treatment or proper nutrition.
- Meet with a group of parents to learn what health information they would like to obtain.

Hints for success:
- Work in collaboration with teachers and parents to identify necessary topics and then develop appropriate interventions.
- Involve graphic design students in the development of printed educational materials.

Site: High School

Theme of clinical assignment: Addressing a health care concern of community adolescents

Design of experience:
    Contact time: 2 hours a week for 10 weeks
    Nursing students: 2–3

Objectives:
    High school students
        Work successfully as a group
        Identify youth's health care concerns for the community
        Collaborate with nursing and medical students
    Nursing students
        Organize a group of high school youth in the community
        Conduct a survey of their health concerns
        Develop a community-based response to a specific need
        Collaborate within an interdisciplinary team

Required supplies/ equipment/ abilities:
    Supplies: paper and writing utensils
    Tools: computer with word processing and graphic arts printing capability
    Abilities of nursing students: lead group process through exploration of concerns
        develop a work plan

provide leadership to complete project
Developmental process:
- Meet with high school guidance counselors to convene group representative of diversity of community
- Work with group to select and define project, develop time line, explore individual expectations

Implementation:
- Set up meeting times and places
- Identify roles for all participants and group leaders
- Identify adolescents' concerns
- Lead group in selection of one and development of a plan to address it.

  Concerned about drug use by younger children, the adolescents decided to develop a drug awareness book for elementary school children. It was community-based, multi-cultural, and literacy appropriate
- Lead iterative process for design of book and consensus process on contents
- Ensure that work is translated appropriately into all languages of community

Evaluation:
- Students demonstrate ability to work in a collaborative process
- Students contribute to the selection and preparation of educational material so that it is age appropriate for expected audience

- Adolescents praise the process of development and the final product
- Elementary children utilize the book appropriately in subsequent educational sessions

Variation on experience:
- Process may be applied to a variety of concerns
- May use TV or newspaper stories as basis of lessons for book
- May ask elementary students to supply stories to use as bases of lessons

Hints for success:
- Prepare nursing students for age appropriate behaviors
- Be alert to possible cultural differences
- Learn from the adolescents the community's cultural makeup and value systems
- Explore with the adolescents helpful techniques to teach about refusing drugs and what to do if they see drugs or drug behaviors

**Site: Homeless shelter for women with substance abuse problems and
their children**
Theme of clinical assignment: Health promotion with mothers
Design of experience:
 Contact time: 2–3 hours for 10 weeks
 Nursing students: 2–3
Objectives:
 For clients
  Identify health care concerns and choose assistance
  Identify parenting concerns and choose assistance
 For nursing students
  Employ interviewing skills.
  Assess actual and potential health problems of adult clients.
  Assess actual or potential health problems of children.
  Apply interventions and referrals as indicated.
Required supplies/ equipment/ abilities:
 Supplies: instructional video tapes and health promotion literature
 Equipment: VCR and television
 Abilities:
  interviewing skills
  diligence in locating and securing educational materials capable of
   planning and implementing both individual and group teaching
Developmental process:
 • Approach the director of a residential facility and offer the assistance
  of students.
 • Explore the potential roles for students and the general concerns of
  the staff for the clientele.
 • Establish goals for the experience that meet the needs of the facility as
  well as the nursing students.
 • Students will be oriented by the staff to the facility and learn from
  them what they perceive to be the health care needs of their clients.
 • Each student will be assigned an identified role within the current
  structure of the facility.
Implementation:
 • Students will work with the women to assess their individual and
  group health care needs.
 • Each student will attempt to develop an individual relationship with
  one family group within the shelter. By talking with the women
  students learned some of the factors that led to their clients'
  present situations.
 • Each student will continue to assess the needs of the group as well as
  their individual client and develop appropriate responses. Students learned from the mothers that they wanted information

about parenting, sexual abuse, AIDS, safe sex and hygiene as well as how to achieve a career in nursing. Some issues were dealt with on an individual basis while others included all clients. Examples of group interventions include workshops on sexual abuse; on parenting skills; and on hygiene, safe sex, and AIDS.

Printed materials, posters, and videotapes were used in the teaching process.

- Assistance will be provided in locating and securing appropriate referrals.

Evaluation:

- Staff express satisfaction of collaborative efforts with students.

- Students demonstrate the ability to interact with clients experiencing multiple difficulties and develop a plan of care that addresses the needs of the group.

- Students demonstrate the ability to interact with clients experiencing multiple difficulties and develop a plan of care that addresses the needs of an individual family.

- Students assess effectiveness of intervention and plan follow-up sessions.

Variation on experience:

- Variation in experience is provided by site specifics. Some sites house only men, others only pregnant women, others only those with AIDS, etc. Expectations of students are geared to the needs of the clients and the level of the students' ability. If a student is assigned to a facility on a repetitive basis the strength of the relatedness to clients increases and as student's nursing abilities increase so too will their role within the facility.

Hints for success:

- Prepare students for the probable indifference and even possible hostility clients may express when a student sits down near them to talk. Help them not to take it as a personal insult but to see it as a learned response to prior events. Developing relationships with these clients may take a great deal of time.

- Provide frequent opportunities for students to talk about their feelings. They may become shaken as they come to know the clients and realize that they are not very different from themselves. Some will be highly educated, some will have jobs, some may be individuals they have previously known.

Site: Senior Center
Theme of clinical assignment: Promoting Health Status—Flu Shot Clinic
Design of experience:

Contact time: 2 hours for 5 weeks

Nursing students: 1 student/ 4 seniors

Objectives:

For senior citizens:

Obtain injection to protect clients from the effects of influenza

Identify possible side effects and describe comfort measures

For nursing students:

Employ skills in planning, advertising, and promoting a community health event.

Apply skills of interviewing, history taking, and injection.

Required supplies/ equipment/ abilities:

Supplies: serum, consent forms, paper goods and printing abilities to make posters

Tools: stethoscope and sphygmomanometer, needles, syringes, alcohol wipes, cotton balls, bandaids

Abilities of nursing students:

take history and screen for appropriateness to receive injection

draw up serum, prepare site and administer serum

monitor client's reaction to serum and provide appropriate teaching

Developmental process:

- Determine the need to make this service available to neighborhood clients.

Implementation:

- Locate a gathering place for senior citizens or a site to which seniors may come.
- Students will estimate the number of clients to be served and arrange to obtain the necessary supplies and doses of vaccine.
- Arrange for availability of emergency transportation if a client requires it due to adverse reaction.
- Develop advertising literature in appropriate languages and reading level.
- Distribute fliers to sites frequented by seniors.
- Spread information through less traditional routes such as church bulletins, pulpit announcements, and community groups.
- Arrange for secondary inducements such as refreshments.
- Consider using the event to distribute health promotion or information concerning health care services to the participants.
- Student cares for a client from intake to discharge: provides teaching and obtains consent for treatment, takes a client history, prepares and administers injection, monitors client for potential adverse reaction, and discharges when process completed.

Evaluation:

- Attendance meets expectations.

- Students demonstrate ability in teaching clients and obtaining informed consent.
- Students demonstrate ability to prepare clients and provide injections.

Value to students:
- By walking through the complete experience with multiple clients, students
  –obtain the chance to do injections repeatedly
  –are able to compare and contrast their nursing intervention abilities with a variety of clients.
- Learn the multiple steps in the process of developing a successful community-based intervention.

Variation on experience:
- Examples of other clinics: childhood immunizations
immunizations for pneumococcal pneumonia
- Clinics such as this may be offered wherever people gather
  –at city airport for taxi drivers
  –after church services
  –at voting sites

Hints for success:
- Learn from community residents when and where the session should be held to obtain the best attendance.
- Involve the community residents and organizations in spreading the word about the session.

Index